I WALKED THAT PATH TOO

COMPILED BY SOPHIE ROUMÉAS

I WALKED THAT PATH TOO
Inspiring stories of resilience.

Copyright ©2023 by Sophie Rouméas

Legal deposit: October 2023

Printed in the United States of America

ISBN 978-2-9578712-0-9
Publisher information:

Angel Lab Editions is a brand and division of
SBR Coaching & Resources
7 rue des Chalets
74940 Annecy Le Vieux, France

DEDICATION

To Christiane-Joséphine, to every author of
this book, to all those we love, who touch our
lives, and inspire us to take up our pens.

To each person who channels energy toward healing,
nurtures the spirit of solidarity and resilience,
utilizes their skills and talents, whether in the
medical field or not, and embraces universal love to
facilitate pacification and healing, from the smallest
individual cell to the grandest collective scale.

We dedicate this book especially to you, the reader, who
may be facing the challenge of breast cancer or caring
for someone who is. Know that we care too, as reflected
in the title of our anthology, 'I Walked That Path Too.'"

ENDORSEMENTS

"*I Walked That Path Too*" is a profoundly moving book, touching the depths of human connection in the face of life's most daunting challenges. With heartfelt gratitude to Sophie for crafting a precious gift for everyone affected by breast cancer. To the courageous women who shared their stories, deep bows of gratitude to you for courageously illuminating the path from tragedy to miracles. Thank you for this invaluable message of perseverance and hope!

Lori Leyden, PhD, MBA

#1 Bestselling Author, Trauma Healing Pioneer, Visionary Spiritual Mentor

Most books on breast cancer focus on the survivor's perspective. It is the most important one. But breast cancer can shatter a much larger reality involving also caretakers, friends, healers, family, doctors, poets... As an exercise of Kintsugi, the Japanese art of repairing, this book carefully brings together the broken parts of a unique story where no one is alone. That is the beauty and the truth we discover in these pages: We are still fighting. Together, as one. We are still here, alive. And that is all that matters. Open this book and listen to all these unbroken voices.

Dr. Maria D. Bermudez

Gender expert, University of California- Irvine.

I read this beautiful anthology in one sitting, but I know that I'll go back and read the chapters again from time to time as women in my practice and in my life - possibly even myself - encounter the path of breast cancer. These personal stories of women who walked this path, as well as contributions from cancer-related family members and caregivers, offer inspiration, practical instruction, and even humor. "I *Walked That Path Too*" is a valuable addition to the growing awareness of breast cancer and, more importantly, how to survive and thrive as a woman who is always so much more than her diagnosis.

Dr. Liz Lyster

DrLizMD.com

President, Rotary Club of Peninsula Starlight 2022-2023

From lyrical poetry to a functional manual, this book is a gift for anyone navigating breast cancer, for yourself or a loved one. There is nothing hypothetical or clinical here. These writings are as raw and personal as stories can be. Some chapters are straight narrative, some internal dialogue, and some dreams. There's even real wisdom from some men who haven't experienced breast cancer, but they know it. Like Gawande's *Being Mortal*, every adult will benefit by reading this marvelous book.

Hedda and Joe DiNucci

aginginterrupted.com

Surrender to love. Healing is a process rooted in love.
—Jane Hutchinson to all the women with breast cancer

TABLE OF CONTENTS

Sophie ROUMÉAS
Introduction

Compassion arises from understanding.
—*Sophie Rouméas*

Note to readers,

Welcome to the caring space of I Walked that Path Too. This book was born from an awareness of the loneliness created by a breast cancer diagnosis. We initiated the anthology as an inspiring companion for a friend, relative, life partner, caregiver, and anyone who wants to understand this ordeal of life even more than their current understanding.

Today, breast cancer is treated better and better than in the past. While millions of women around the world live the challenge of breast cancer, its prevention has been refined and scaled across the population. National and international authorities are allied to stabilize and reduce the cases of women (and men[1]) affected by this cancer, and traditional and unconventional medicines have combined with various therapies to take care of each woman in her holistic dimension.

---

[1] 1% of men develop breast cancer in the world according to the World Health Organization.

Many women who receive a breast-cancer diagnosis feel as though their lives have been turned upside down. Cancer touches women's bodies at the heart of the cells, many times hidden from awareness for years; but their conscience, their emotions, are hit hard in the precise moment of the revelation of the disease. Their world changes dimension and priorities. There is a "before" and an "after" diagnosis. Even though women may receive medical information immediately and have adequate physical and emotional support, there are often moments of great loneliness experienced by them and their loved ones.

My name is Sophie Rouméas and without having had breast cancer myself, I kept in my heart the indelible and discreet trace of my aunt's disease until the day when I understood that she had found her way to give meaning to her experience and that it was my turn to share in solidarity with her.

My paternal aunt, Christiane-Joséphine, lived 96 years. Diagnosed with breast cancer approaching her fifty years in the early 80s, she was treated physically with the removal of the affected breast. I was barely ten years old at that time, and despite the precautions taken by the adults in my family, I caught snippets of conversations about my aunt's state of health that shocked me. "They will have to remove her breast" was engraved in my childhood memory like an inconceivable mutilation. The lively words overheard while passing when I was a child, became verified when, as a teenager during a summer stay at her house, I saw my aunt placing small malleable pockets in her bra in place of breasts. At that time, breast reconstructions were not as available as they are now. For this reason, among others, my aunt would have benefited from receiving experienced psychological support, but this was still only partially included in the care pathways.

Despite a soulful sadness that I could sometimes feel in her, and even if this period of her life disengaged her from her love life, her partner, my aunt nevertheless subsequently lived as peaceful a life as she could. She transcended her dreams and hopes by expressing them in her creations of shimmering, uplifting, and inspired silk paintings. She gave meaning to her experience and recreated her own value by sharing her art.

Aunt Christiane-Joséphine transitioned as she lived, gracefully and serenely, this spring of 2023. I pay homage that she instilled the grace, order, and beauty of her soul into her discreet and artistic nature. Through her attitude, she taught me softness in the face of adversity, patience in the face of illness, acceptance of what is, and art as a powerful form of resilience.

Nine out of ten women are cured of breast cancer for five years or more according to the World Health Organization and the current global statistics. This is one of the best cancer survival rates in the world today. However, breast cancer is still the leading cause of cancer death in women today; though, health authorities estimate that one in eight women will develop breast cancer in her lifetime, and developing countries as well as minorities need much more prevention, early detection, and access to treatment. The fact that positive progression has been made should not prevent us from continuing to understand, support and care for families who walk the path of cancer.

Because of this reality, all healing actors have mobilized to improve patient care. The physical condition being the first impacted by the disease, as soon as the cancer is detected, everything is put in place to contain, then eradicate, the affected cells and organs. The more we advance in time, the more the other human dimensions are considered. It is now common for a woman who has been diagnosed with cancer to be offered a list of multidisciplinary practices and associations for the purpose of psychological, emotional, and spiritual support. This is a positive evolution. Even if we do not quantitatively measure the positive impact of psychological and psychosomatic monitoring, it is recognized today that the quality of resilience of the people who benefit from it is improved.

Through the intimate stories and inspiring quotes shared in this book, we invite you to encounter the existence of a capacity for truth. The "capacity for truth" was first coined by the French physician Christian Tal Schaller as part of his holistic medicine and healing approach. It refers to the belief in the inherent ability of the body to heal and rebalance itself when obstacles to health are removed; this is in the interest of any person affected by the disease, and to their care team, to build and maintain over time the physical and psychological resources that help them overcome their disease and to regain their own value.

Through the breast cancer journey, the vulnerability that invites itself into the emotional sphere of the patients fragilizes them, but as Professor Cynthia Fleury[2] points out, "It can also be the occasion for a possible sublimation, which moreover often is, as the individual regains his individuation in the light of the existential trials he is going through. Reading the lives of creators often reveals the pangs they experienced before transforming themselves into style, art, work, progress, and knowledge for the rest of mankind."

---

[2] Cynthia Fleury, philosopher and psychoanalyst, author of the book *Le soin est un humanisme* (*Care is a humanism*), published by Gallimard, for whom "*it is so important to make each individual 'capable', that is to say capable of relationship and self-sovereignty.* »

Therefore, we have humbly compiled the chapters of this book as testimonies of encouragement for those who have received the diagnosis of cancer.

You will thus read unique stories told by amazing storytellers ... women who have lived through the ordeal of breast cancer and share their personal path to healing; in another chapter, a young woman, describes how she navigated the challenge of her mother's illness to her recovery. Also, four proficient therapists committed beyond international borders bring their support and awareness to the cause, and a poet expresses his solidarity by lending his voice to full presence. Their narratives reveal facets of humanity, such as doubt, encouragement, fear, faith, willpower, inspiration, resilience, acceptance, compassion, dignity, femininity, love, knowledge, transformation ... The path to healing can also be a source of profound changes and metamorphoses towards a renewed life. The physical experience of cancer, the medical journey that follows, is intimately linked to emotions, reflection, intention, awareness, and solidarity.

On a planet where a billion human beings live, each ordeal of life invites sharing. May its burden be lightened to those who carry it.

- Sophie Rouméas, Angel Lab Editions.

Crystal Weber

The sound of remission

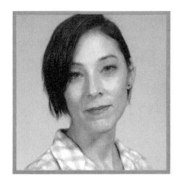 A writer at heart, Crystal Weber works as a translator and interpreter from French and Spanish into English. She was born in California and currently lives in France. She has always been passionate about dance and more recently yoga. She finds her inspiration in the glimmers of her daily experience.

Crystal fell ill with breast cancer in 2018 and has now been in remission for four years. Her experience with illness pushed her on a quest to get to know her real self and to heal. For this, yoga has been an essential tool. In 2020, she completed a yoga teacher training programme and has been teaching hatha flow yoga classes on the side for two years.

Currently, she is enrolled in a yoga therapy course and in the future aims to offer one-on-one consultations to help people heal and find peace in their lives regardless of what ails them. She would also like to focus on supporting cancer patients during and after their treatments through yoga therapy.

To find out more about Crystal, visit: www.crystalnicole weber.com

Crystal Weber
The sound of remission

Don't ask what the world needs. Ask
what makes you come alive and go
do it. Because what the world needs
is people who have come alive.
—Howard Thurman

Remission.

Remission rings with submission, intermission, prohibition...

Four years of remission

but tumors continue to haunt and taunt me

into decomposition.

They appear in my dreams and when I wake,

I check my body to make sure, rest assured,

phew, it's not a premonition.

They appear in trees, bulging from the side of their trunks

in an inconsiderate show of bedazzlement.

In the off-kilter walls of quaint Parisian apartments

just begging to be photographed.

In that imperfect zucchini
rejected, dejected, and tossed into the half-off bin
in a plea to save the planet.

And then the worst of all,
they pop up in the people around me: my ex-father in law's
liver, in the brain of a friend-once-removed,
in a former colleague's breast,
in my grandfather's colon,
in my dog's snout.

You see?
They are everywhere, always lurking about.

Remission also rings with drought.
My body hasn't seen rain in six months.
My insides are unexpectedly lit ablaze,
rampant wildfires with no regard for place or time,
during a presentation at work, a pirouette on stage,
an al fresco dinner with friends, or in the dead of night...

Despite the moisturizers, deep repair creams and serums,
the skin on my face grows tight,

and the desert gains ground,

turning old fertile stomping grounds into dust strewn vacant
lots,

where no one wants to play

on the broken swings for fear of getting hurt

on the rusty metal parts that threaten to fall apart

at the slightest touch.

Knock knock.

My boyfriend asks to be let in anyway.

He wants to play

on the playground

despite the drought.

Remission also rings with numbness.

The refusal of certain body parts to register textures and sensations

but also the will not to feel

the sting of words

when lovers say, "Why are your breasts so cold? I don't like touching them,"

when ex-husbands say, "Everyone is replaceable,"

when friends say, "Don't worry, everything will be alright,"

when doctors say, "At your age, it's about time for an ovariectomy,"

when mothers say, "Talking won't change the past,"

when colleagues say, "When are you going to get serious and have a baby?"

when bosses say, "You must obey the rules, just like everyone else," when I finally stand up and say, "No. I'm not like everyone else."

And the expectations of others crumble and tumble

cascading down around me in dangerous shards of broken glass.

Good thing my feet are numb

and can walk on broken glass.

Remission also rings with duty,

day in and day out,

despite the meaningless motions,

playing the part of a cog in a machine

I neither invented nor convened.

My heart says this is not the way

but my mind says, yes, it is because it pays.

What they have decided is reality

does not interest me,

and so I take refuge in my wildest reveries.

A place full of gentle giant plants who speak poetry.

Where humans and flowers bow to each other in mutual respect

of each other's most perfect worth.

But then my phone vibrates

and it's back to work.

Remission also rings with fear
of overexertion
of rejection
of loneliness
of not having the resources
of not being enough
of not keeping up
of not knowing what my body
is capable of

of lightning striking twice in the same spot...

Comforting lap of denial, please hold me for a little bit longer.
Tell me how
it can't be me, I've done my time,
how the universe is on my side,
even though statistics say otherwise.
When the numbers add up,
Science has spoken,
and we all know
that her sentence cannot be broken.
The birds chirping in the morning
awake me from my restless slumber.

They say, "My dear.

"Listen to our song of ancient traditions.

"Listen

"as we sing it for all to hear."

Remission also rings with wisdom,

the lessons I should have learned,

blah blah blah.

Don't fall victim to victimhood.

Please just let me cry it out without trying to fix

something that was not broken to begin with.

The constant duality of the world:

Good vs. bad,

Me vs. you,

Me vs. the world,

Me vs. me.

In the spaces between the debris,

the contours of my body become clear,

surrounded by a silver lining.

I now see where I stop and you begin.

The quiver of a lip,

the contraction of the inner thigh,

the tightness of the throat,

the nausea in the gut,

they all mean "NO.

"Danger, watch out.

"Not here, not now.

"Please, slow down."

The body speaks before words have a chance to be born,

but who would listen to the unborn?

Remission also rings with confusion.

The wily disguises of my mind,

always tricking me into believing that I'm less than this

or no more than that.

If left to root will uproot

the delicate seedlings of faith and trust that I have planted deep within,

who are nourished by the light of that subtle voice,

the one that knows before I know,

the sun cannot be risen before dawn.

Time and time again

I become blind

to what is simple and true.

Nothing ever existed.

Never will.

I WALKED THAT PATH TOO

All is just as it is,
without a ring in its bell.

Yet the mind
will go on touting its tune,
but this time
I will take heed
of the lyrics I write.

Remission rings with transmission, permission, fruition.
Do you hear it?
Just sit still...
and listen.

Dr Lopamudra Das Roy

Save a life, save a family

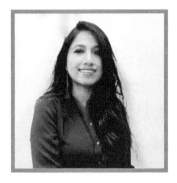

Dr. Lopamudra Das Roy, cancer research professor and social entrepreneur, founded Breast Cancer Hub in 2017 with a dream to save lives at no cost to patients or families by making impactful and sustainable changes at the grassroots level and by bridging the gap between the developed and developing worlds. Breast Cancer Hub is a GuideStar Platinum Certified, top-rated 501 (c)(3) nonprofit organization registered in North Carolina, USA.

Dr. Das Roy has twenty-two-plus years of experience in research, teaching, and mentoring undergraduate and PhD candidates in the field of genetics and cancer. She has a PhD in genetics (molecular biology) from India, post-doctoral fellowship from Mayo Clinic College of Medicine, and an MBA from Northwestern University-Kellogg School of Management. She served at University of North Carolina, Charlotte, as research professor, was awarded grants from the Department of Defense as principal investigator for the cancer research program and National Cancer Institute and investigated targeted therapies and signaling pathways in cancer. She is recognized as a Distinguished Cancer Scientist with high-impact publications, inventions, citations, and press releases from the American Association of Cancer Research for breakthrough work on discovering the signaling pathway between breast cancer metastasis and arthritis.

Dr. Das Roy has received many global awards, but the greatest happiness comes from bringing smiles to the families of innumerable lives she saves each day in the urban and rural areas in utmost need, who would have otherwise gone undetected. She has dedicated her life to the purpose of humanity, serving the community and patients.

Lopamudra, MS, Ph.D., MBA, Founder and President, Breast Cancer Hub

Email: lopa@breastcancerhub.org, lopa2006@gmail.com

Website: https://www.breastcancerhub.org/

LinkedIn: https://www.linkedin.com/in/lopamudradasroy/

Dr Lopamudra Das Roy
Save a life, save a family

Each of us makes a difference
- Together We Save Lives.
—Dr Lopa

Growing up, I cannot remember a single day when my father and grandfather didn't discuss a challenging medical issue at our dinner table. My father, a pediatrician, advocated for "breast milk," and I was oblivious, until I was twelve years old when one of my friends' mothers passed away, that the word "breast" was associated with stigma and taboo. At the funeral, I tried finding the cause of death. To my surprise, people hesitated to mention the word "cancer" and hushed me up when I repeated the words, "**breast cancer.**" I was shocked and questioned, is this the respect we give to a mother who lost her life, that we can't discuss the disease that took it?

The pain of that day stayed within me and I realized how cancer became a household name and death sentence. I wanted to understand the etiology of cancer, to discover the pathways to cure and treatment therapy, and to educate society about the concept of early detection and preventable measures so that death rates were reduced worldwide.

Growing up in India, I witnessed the suffering of cancer patients and how cancer can ruin one family in just a few months if not detected early. My heart sank when I saw young lives taken due to late detection of breast cancer; the death rate being significantly higher in the developing world. I discussed with breast cancer patients/advocates from the USA the pain and agony when mammograms failed their diagnoses due to dense breast tissues.

Currently, worldwide, breast cancer in men is increasing and most men with breast cancer seem to experience shock and embarrassment, battling the "stigma" of having a predominantly woman's disease. Similarly, the LGBTQ+ community is facing extreme challenges from the healthcare screening and treatment standpoint. As a cancer research professor and principal investigator, my heart questioned over the years if we were also addressing the fundamental challenges that could shift the paradigm of the healthcare system and save lives in underprivileged areas where there is no one to take care of them. Women, men, and LGBTQ+ have lost their lives to breast and other cancers due to taboo, ignorance, lack of awareness leading to late detection, inaccessibility to healthcare facilities, inaccurate diagnoses, and poor treatment management.

In 2017, I was determined to build Breast Cancer Hub (BCH), but it would not be easy because commitments would be beyond family and health. My personal life was rough with chronic health challenges. After seven miscarriages, God bestowed me with two miracle babies in 2010 and 2011. I knew that to execute sustainable changes in developing countries, I had to leave my young kids and travel to remote sectors on my own in public commutes, risking my safety. But it was a calling. I resigned from my job and created BCH, a global community, standing against discrimination of color, religion, language, culture, and gender, using slogans, such as #BreakTheCancerTaboo, #KnowYourBody, #TogetherWeSavelives, and #BreakTheBreastTaboo, which brought huge criticism from conservative sectors. But I remained stern and undeterred.

I dedicated my life to fighting breast cancer in women, men, and the LGBTQ+ community, as well as supporting the fight against all types of cancers, via BCH Wings, Cancer Hubs, with the goals of: 1) raising awareness and focusing on education, early detection, and prevention; 2) researching at the grassroots level; 3) creating community outreaches, analyzing reports, navigating suspicious cases towards healthcare facilities, finding affordable options and taking accountability; 4) organizing screening camps; 5) adopting villages (BCH is the pioneer) for door-to-door cancer screening, diagnosis, treatment aid and management, and palliative care; 6) forming patient support groups; 7) holding medical guidance and patient counseling (one-on-one); 8) creating patient-care packages, including mastectomy or lumpectomy comfort pillows with a pocket that holds a cold or hot pack for healing, knitted chemo hats, and chemo port seat-belt pillows; 9) devising pandemic and flood response; 10) creating leadership mentorship programs to train next-generation leaders in healthcare.

BCH stands apart as a cancer organization by creating a unique model where all our services are free and 100 percent of donations from kindhearted supporters are driven toward our mission. Every day is challenging, but our work speaks volumes, as we accomplish goals by improvising, based on the circumstances and needs of the community, keeping the vision and mission intact with our core values—ethics, integrity, and transparency.

The road is hard when our vision is to revolutionize and uproot the fundamental stigmas imbibed in our society over the years. In developing countries, a huge population is stricken by poverty, with healthcare being the last priority. In the USA, many minority communities delay early-detection screening processes due to the inherent culture of disregard for breast health, leading to late detection and death. Therefore, I fight not only the rural populace's poor access to the hospital system, but also urban society's inertia to discuss breast concerns due to ingrained ideology of shyness about breast health.

Breast cancer is increasing in the younger populace of all genders, especially the high-risk population. Therefore, if symptoms are noticed for any gender, immediate attention should be taken and reported to a doctor.

Another area that needs attention is ground research. The lack of global clinical data on breast cancer across demographics and cultures, especially from the developing world, bothers me. This critical situation will not be taken seriously until and unless we understand the status and frequency of cancer, collectively, in cities and villages (remote) through appropriate data collection and analysis. We must decode the determinants that cause the advancement of non-metastatic breast cancer into metastatic Stage 4, shedding light on the biological and circumstantial factors affecting progression and investigating the incidence in diverse age groups, ethnicities, and younger populations. We must bridge the gap between the developed and developing worlds to uplift the research potential and bring to light the current situation of breast cancer and other types of cancer in the urban and rural sectors across the globe and try to decipher the hidden elements that may eventually help in the treatment schema and change the healthcare policies.

BCH's biggest challenge evolved while executing our mission in the adopted villages for door-to-door cancer screening, diagnosis, treatment management, palliative care, and counselling. We learned that food was the priority for the villagers and that they rarely saw the face of hospitals. The villagers were daily wage earners, living a hand-to-mouth existence without any savings. On many occasions, there was no one in the family to accompany the patient to the hospital, eventually delaying or skipping treatment. Therefore, BCH takes full responsibility, starting from providing transport, accompanying patients to local hospitals that provide treatment at subsidized rates, assisting with hospital registration and patient-doctor communication, helping in generating the income certificate to help patients access the government-aided schemes, assisting in the full screening and diagnosis process, buying necessary medicines, providing treatment aid for the remaining expenses not covered under the government schemes, and returning them home with follow-ups and counseling. The recent pandemic built new challenges in the villages we adopted, but poverty needs to be addressed in a holistic manner, and we addressed this by distributing masks and sanitizers, generating safety protocols, providing food relief, and taking care, end to end.

When diagnosed with cancer, it is not just about the patient but also the family. The emotional turmoil is profound, along with societal myths that come along. We need to bring comfort, care, and compassion to the families and hold hands on the journey, providing them with the correct scientific information and medical guidance on treatment. In a village in India in 2018, I met a young mother, fighting advanced Stage 4 breast cancer. She lived in a small mud house, and I was shocked to find her lying on the floor on a thin bed sheet. The family was scared to touch her stating that "cancer is contagious." I helped her to the bed and explained to the family that cancer is not contagious, that a cancer patient needs love and affection. After ages, her kids hugged her, and though she was in excruciating pain, she looked at me and gave a priceless smile because now she would leave this world in the arms of her family. This was my precious reward.

It is heartbreaking to come across many similar instances of patients facing isolation when diagnosed with cancer, even in the diverse ethnic cultures across developed and developing countries, irrespective of education and socio-economic condition. A common statement I hear is, "Dr. Lopa, please do not add me to your BCH support group because I want to remain anonymous, or my daughters will not get married." Only five to ten percent of all cancer cases occur due to inherited genetic mutations. The remaining ninety to ninety-five percent have their roots in the environment, lifestyle, or occur randomly. It is our responsibility to translate the information to the community, and even if we fall in the five- to ten-percent category, we can take precautionary measures and perform screening earlier than the recommended age.

Breast cancer, when detected early and treated accurately, is curable. Breast cancer screening is the key, which means looking for signs before a person has symptoms, helping to find cancer at an early stage, with better survival, which will bring a positive shift; but the healthcare system must provide avenues to help patients who are uninsured or can't afford treatment due to financial crisis, which is the sustainable solution.

Paths of Breast Cancer Screening

- Breast Self-Exam (BSE): Starting at the age of seventeen to eighteen years and understanding the look and feel of our breasts—any abnormalities, any discharges, any painless or painful lump. *If any of these symptoms occur,* please immediately reach out to us or contact your healthcare system. BCH generated BSE cards in twenty-four languages for all genders. Please download, share, and save lives at https://www.breastcancerhub. org/news-2/self-breast-exam-card

- Clinical breast exam, an examination of the breast by a doctor or nurse.

- Mammogram screening after the age of forty. Mammograms may miss about half of cancers with dense breast, therefore, supplemental tests—3D mammogram/tomosynthesis, breast ultrasound, breast MRI/MBI—are needed as per a doctor's guidance.

- High-risk population, please check early.

Here's a one-stop card with breast cancer screening information: https://www.breastcancerhub.org/educational -cards/breastcancer-screening

Below, I share a few stories from the community as they opened to me, which helps us understand that raising awareness requires more than screening; it needs a holistic approach.

- "Wish I knew a painless lump I felt all along was cancer, then I wouldn't have been diagnosed at end stage."

- "I got diagnosed with breast cancer at the age of twenty-eight. I was about to get married to the love of my life, but my would-be in-laws broke my marriage. I am thirty-eight now, a survivor, but I stopped believing in love and marriage."

- "I am a son and a doctor, but I never asked my mother to go for breast cancer screening, and she was always shy to discuss the lump in her breast. My mother is on her deathbed now."

- "A male doctor examined my breast and asked me to come back to the hospital for an ultrasound. I never went back as I was so embarrassed and didn't want any other male doctor to touch my breast. Now I am at advanced metastatic breast cancer."

- "I am a male breast-cancer patient. My kids at school are hesitant to disclose my breast cancer, as their friends will bully them, as it's a woman's disease."

- "I have a family history, but my diagnosis was delayed as there is no screening mammogram for the males."

- "Being a male, I do not want to wear a pink gown for my diagnostic mammogram. Can we have a blue gown please? Men have breasts too."

- "Why didn't you come to my village last year? My forty-two-year-old mother just died. She didn't know the symptoms of breast cancer, and due to shyness, didn't tell anyone."

These stories are just a small group of the eye-opening instances reported to me.

In today's world, advancement has touched our lives with technology, science, and medicine, yet our MIND preaches the stigma engulfing our society for ages. Love, care, affection, and the feeling of togetherness are what families need. I have created support groups with patients, survivors, oncologists, caregivers, and nurses, sharing expertise and life experiences, with immense emotional bonding, standing for each other. My one-on-one time with patients is my moment of satisfaction as I help scientifically guide and counsel them through the process. We publish incredible journeys of cancer thrivers in local languages, providing strength to others fighting cancer. We honor cancer thrivers and the lives departed with the "BCH-The Bravest Hero Award," carrying the legacy of the brave-hearts, as our cancer fighters are our heroes!

I believe: We Save a Life, We Save a Family!

Inès Martin

Abandoned memories

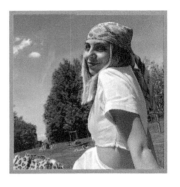

I'm Inès and I am student in international business in France. My life is punctuated by university, sports, my student job and my family (including my boyfriend) with whom I share a lot of time.

My story is the one I lived through with my mom's cancer. I hope you'll be able to find yourself through my words, or simply that my experience will help you if you're going through this moment.

The thing to know: I wrote this chapter from the heart.

Contact Inès at Inès Martin | LinkedIn

www.linkedin.com/in/inès-martin

Inès Martin
Abandoned memories

*Life is not about waiting for the
storm to pass. It's about learning
how to dance in the rain.*
—Seneca

I was fifteen years old when I learned, through a phone call from my mom as she came out of a doctor's appointment, that she had been diagnosed with that dreaded illness: breast cancer. Learning and trying to understand my mother's diagnosis was quite a challenge for me.

At fifteen, torn between anger and sadness amidst the turmoil of adolescence, I held a grudge against the world and carried a chip on my shoulder. I didn't know how to handle the situation. I struggled to show my emotions and feelings that I kept bottled up regarding the situation. I shut down rather than reaching out to my mom, having conversations to learn more about her illness, taking care of her, and truly being there as a support and a shoulder to lean on. In hindsight, I think I was afraid to truly grasp what she was going through and how much she might be suffering with the heavy treatments and the changes they bring in physical appearance.

A week has passed since I wrote the above. During the week between, I took the time to discuss what I had already written with my grandmother, whom I am very close to, in the hope of unearthing memories from that period, which has been taboo for me and appears as a void in my mind. The first thing she told me was that, contrary to my memory, it wasn't my mom who had told me about her illness, but rather my father. Indeed, after my grandmother's words, I was confused and quite lost, because in my few remaining memories, I thought at least this one was correct. At that moment, she also added that I had never accepted my mom's illness and that I was filled with anger. This is where I questioned my ability to write this chapter because, without memories, it's hard to talk about the past and my experience. And then I did some research and concluded: My brain had developed a defense mechanism to erase traumatic and painful memories. I did, though, hold on to one memory, perhaps not in detail, but I think it's important to mention.

When my mom started her chemotherapy, I understood that she was going to undergo physical changes. I knew she would lose weight, which frightened me a bit because with her slender build, her healthy weight was 43 kilograms (about 95 pounds). When you lose weight from 43 kilograms, the difference becomes noticeable quite quickly. But the thing that hurt me the most was the thought of her losing her hair. I dreaded that moment, I think out of fear of truly grasping the situation beyond what I was already aware of. At first, she wore a small cap at home to prevent me from seeing her hairless scalp. And what remains etched in my memory is the day I went to visit her at the clinic with my father. I felt at that precise moment, after some time, that it was okay for me to see her without her hair, and that ultimately, the apprehension I had was unwarranted because she was still the same person and just as beautiful.

Certainly, if I had been the teenager in the body of the young woman I am now, I wouldn't have reacted in the same way, but this event in my life is part of what made me who I am. It made me grow, mature, put things into perspective, change. That's why both the negative and positive aspects of how I reacted and thought at that time are a part of my story.

With time and the passing years, I've been able to reflect on what happened to my mom and, ultimately, on myself as well. I wonder if I could have been as strong and resilient if I were in her place, if I could have focused only on the positive, seen myself without hair without despising myself, endured exhausting treatments, supported myself with one less breast that takes away a part of my femininity.

Femininity holds significant meaning for many women, certainly for me. It's synonymous with physical and mental well-being, with a flourishing presence in society. That's why realizing that breast cancer can take away certain aspects of femininity is a heart-wrenching ordeal. But precisely, every woman is beautiful with her differences, and that's what gives the power and authenticity to each one.

If I ever have a conversation with a little girl who learns that her mom has breast cancer, I would tell her not to be afraid. Fear is what draws us into denial of a situation, as I did with my mom's illness, which plunged me into a complete refusal to accept reality.

If you resonate with fear, anger, and sadness, you'll resist facing the reality of the situation you're in and the presence you'll need to have. On the other hand, if you resonate with hope and positivity, you'll move towards the path of acceptance, where you'll be needed to spread goodness and offer your support.

Acceptance becomes the key to moving forward; although for me, it wasn't at all spontaneous or obvious. When faced with this situation, we need to embrace the new reality as it is, without trying to control or deny it, because in this trial, every mom needs comfort from her child and anyone else, not negative states.

I would also tell this little girl to talk with her mom to understand everything that's happening and everything that will happen in the months ahead. I would tell her to accompany her mom to her chemotherapy sessions, if she can, something I regret not having done. I would tell her to spend more time with her mom during this time when she might feel weakened and emotionally tested, to provide distractions, to help and encourage her to fight and overcome.

And as a young woman, I would like to remind all of you who are reading this of the vital importance of taking care of ourselves and our health. Breast cancer screening is an act of self-love, both for yourself and for those who care about you. Give yourself this time, your health deserves all the attention you can give it.

To conclude this chapter dedicated to my personal experience, I want to express my admiration for my mom's battle, not only a triumphant one but one that has equipped her with immense strength and positivity in every situation, while it's sincere to say that I would have wished to be present in a different way.

If you're reading this: Kudos, Mom. I love you.

I also want to pay tribute to those women who are currently waging a fierce fight against cancer. Your resilience and strength deserve to be acknowledged. To those who have conquered these challenges with unwavering determination and triumphed like warriors, your story is a source of inspiration for all those facing the same disease. To every woman going through this trial, know that you are not alone. Your courage inspires, your resilience lights the path for others, and your victory offers hope. You are more than just a survivor; you are a beacon of light for all who have the privilege of knowing you.

May this acknowledgment bring a smile to your faces and a glimmer of optimism to your hearts. You are heroes, and your stories deserve to be told with pride.

My thoughts are with you.

In the end, we can endure much
more than we think.
—Frida Kahlo

Joelle Gropper-Kaufman

You Are the Co-Pilot

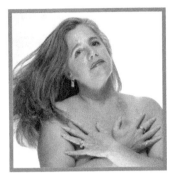

Joelle Gropper Kaufman is an executive coach, revenue catalyst, speaker, and facilitator. She is a transformational leader who teaches leadership practices to sales, marketing, and customer-success executives at Pavilion University. She has worked with individuals, teams, and companies to accelerate growth, become more agile, and creatively address any situation—achieving and sustaining "flow."

Joelle is passionate about leadership, accountability, and innovation. She has spent her adult life exploring leadership and group dynamics and has emerged uniquely skilled in the art of getting stuff done. She has applied that art to her personal (and successful) journey through breast cancer in 2023, as well as her career as a 25+-year sales and marketing executive, and her family, as a wife, mother of three (almost grown) children, and family-by-choice (friends).

Joelle has a BA from the University of Michigan and a MBA from the Harvard Business School where she was a Baker Scholar. She enjoys being with people she loves, traveling, reading, singing (she fronts a rock band), and learning.

joelle@gtmflow.com

www.linkedin.com/in/joellekaufman

www.gtmflow.com

Joelle Gropper-Kaufman
You Are the Co-Pilot

Don't believe what your eyes are telling you. All they show is limitation. Believe with your understanding, find out what you already know, and you'll see the way to fly.
—Richard Bach, Jonathan Livingston Seagull

I was thirteen years old when I first began preparing to face breast cancer. My mother (a thirty-nine-year survivor), sister (a twenty-year survivor), and I all carry the BRCA1 gene. Knowing my genetic probability was eighty percent for breast cancer and forty percent for ovarian cancer, I was proactive about my health—still am. I vigorously exercise, don't smoke, drink infrequently, maintain a low-sugar and low-processed food healthy diet, and get either a mammogram/ultrasound or a bi-lateral MRI every six months. At thirty-eight, I had my ovaries and fallopian tubes removed which brought my ovarian cancer risk below five percent and my breast cancer risk to forty percent.

After a scare at fifty-one, I elected to have a prophylactic bi-lateral mastectomy and DIEP flap reconstruction. During the preliminary scans, one day before surgery, I was diagnosed with a 9mm triple negative fast-growing breast cancer. While there had been no evidence of cancer in my June MRI or in the pathology from my October breast reduction in preparation for the mastectomy and reconstruction, the tumor had spread to a lymph node—making me Stage 2A. I was thankful for early detection, a likely positive response to treatment, and a clear surgical path. I felt confident that, like my sister and mother, I would be a breast cancer survivor.

Instead of having surgery first, my treatment plan included a twelve-week course of Taxol-Carboplatin, one year of Keytruda every three weeks, and an MRI at week eleven or twelve to determine how the tumor was responding. If the response was good but incomplete, I'd have four cycles of Adriamycin and cisplatin (Red Devil) bi-weekly, then the bilateral mastectomy with immediate DIEP flap reconstruction I was supposed to have had in January. I was lucky. My tumor responded to the Taxol-Carbo and my surgery was on May 4, after which I was declared to have a pathological complete response.

Six Steps

Having lived through the experience twice as a family member and once as a patient, I've learned to be a proactive co-pilot with my medical team. The following six steps turned my experience into something loving, generous, and even amusing.

1. Tell everyone

Sharing my diagnosis with my three children (ages twenty-one, nineteen, and sixteen at the time) was the hardest part of the beginning. Despite my full confidence that I would survive, the oxygen left the room when I told them. They knew my family's breast cancer experiences and genetic mutation. They had lived through my mother's recovery from bladder cancer. Each child reacted in accordance with their unique personalities. I invited them to ask questions, express their fears and concerns, and do whatever they needed to do to process. I told them that it was all right if they felt fear for me AND for themselves as this was a genetic cancer. I reminded them that I had been in their shoes as the child of a cancer patient and would support them as best I could. Finally, I asked them to live their lives—focus on school, athletics, music, job searches—whatever was already their top priority; their efforts and stories would distract and elevate me during the treatment marathon. Having been a teenager with a mom going through cancer treatment, I suggested they "tell everyone." At a minimum, I told them to tell people they hoped would support them when things get tough.

Why tell everyone? Because you don't know what others have experienced and support comes from surprising places. When I was diagnosed with breast cancer, it felt as if the world shifted beneath my feet. It's an emotional whirlwind and understandable to want to retreat into yourself. However, sharing the news with your community is crucial in co-piloting your breast cancer experience.

My daughter told people the next day. She discovered that one of her closest friends had lived through her mother's cancer treatment four years earlier. The friend offered my daughter a supportive shoulder. The school advocate offered to communicate with teachers, coaches, and counselors so my daughter wouldn't have to repeat herself. She ultimately made my diagnosis very public by organizing a two-day, eight-team awareness fundraiser for lacrosse teams to "Play for Pink" and raise $4,000 for Sharsheret, a breast cancer research and support organization.

Treatment brings ups and downs, setbacks and surprises. You don't know when you will need compassion from others. Sharing my journey lightened the weight on me and my caregivers' shoulders. My friends and family offered their love, encouragement, and practical assistance. I never felt alone in my journey and letting others in made a big difference.

2. Use CaringBridge to manage who, what, and when people know about your cancer

CaringBridge removed the need for me to repeatedly explain to friends and family what was happening with my delayed surgery, diagnosis, treatment plan, and prognosis. Keeping everyone updated, individually, with their questions, concerns, and well-intentioned curiosity can be exhausting and time-consuming.

CaringBridge allows you to create a webpage to keep your community informed. Users have complete control over what to share and when. A webpage eliminates the need for repeated updates, sparing the emotional energy of recounting the same details repeatedly. Multiple authors contributed to my CaringBridge—myself, my husband, and my BFF, Jessica. It provided an outlet, without obligation, for me to connect and conserved a lot of energy for those helping me.

Through CaringBridge, I empowered my community to stay connected and engaged in a way that suited them. My community received updates, left messages of support, and signed-up to help as they wished. This way, my care team and I focused on my treatment and recovery rather than fielding inquiries.

Though I shared, I chose not to share on social media and asked others to respect that choice. While Facebook can be a wonderful tool for staying connected, it may not be the best platform for sharing the intimate details of a breast cancer journey. Facebook's algorithms and advertising practices can sometimes be less than sensitive.

Remember, co-piloting your breast cancer experience is about empowering yourself. I decided who knew what, how much, and when. By using platforms like CaringBridge and considering the nuances of social media, I navigated this challenging journey with greater ease and maintained my privacy while still receiving the support and love I needed.

3. Be an effective and relentless advocate for your care

Buckle up. I wasn't just a passenger on this breast cancer journey; I was the co-pilot. Adopting a warm, respectful, and active self-advocacy approach was crucial in navigating my way through treatment.

Trust your medical team, but don't hesitate to switch gears if the need arises. TAKE NOTES. In fact, I took someone to major appointments with me to take notes, ensure I heard everything, and list questions to ask. I even used an AI transcription app called "Otter.ai."

Stay vigilant. Question anything that seems amiss. Share everything with your medical team. No detail is irrelevant. Keep accurate records. I have a Google Sheets workbook with different sheets—care team, phone numbers and emails; drain output; symptoms, medication schedule, any reactions; cannabis journal (for nausea or dampening steroid jitters). I don't recommend doing Google searches on protocols and outcomes unless you are medically technical. Outcomes are population-based and don't apply to your individual situation. If you don't trust your treatment team, find a different team.

The following game plan helped me co-pilot my journey: After the first meeting with my care team (my co-pilots), I created a cancer obliteration calendar on Google with essential dates, appointments, and milestones to get a clearer picture of what lay ahead. I used repeating appointments for labs and chemo infusions. I knew that plans may change, but having a comprehensive overview helped me maintain my focus and knowing where the finish line could be alleviated a lot of anxiety. I shared my cancer obliteration calendar with my husband, children, extended family, and BFF[3].

During that first meeting with my care team, I asked for a port. Chemotherapy is toxic and I was sure my veins would not like it. A port is an extra procedure—interventional radiology—but it's quick. The port is used for labs, blood draws, and infusions. I named mine "Voldeport." I advocated for her placement to be a little lower on my chest so that she wasn't highly visible and didn't impair mobility in my shoulder. She's pretty awesome. Once I recovered from her installation, I had no discomfort with Voldeport and had been safeguarded from weekly punctures and vein damage.

One of my fears was long bouts of vomiting. So, in order not to dread this side effect of chemotherapy, I tackled it head-on. Effective anti-nausea medicines, like Emend and Cinvanti, Zofran, Ativan, and Compazine, ensure a queasy-free journey. Cinvanti was my must-have (Emend had helped my sister) and I asked for it in that first meeting and double checked during my first infusion that I was getting it.

Co-piloting and calendar management meant that I had the clearest view of all my appointments—and found that I could manage them to my benefit. I looked out for long

---

[3] BFF stands for "Best Friends Forever".

waiting times, last minute rescheduling, or overlapping bookings. Cancer is a multi-specialty treatment experience—you may have oncology, infusion, breast surgery, plastic surgery, genetic counseling, nutrition, interventional radiology, radiation oncology, and psycho-oncology. Stay organized and don't hesitate to advocate to rearrange things for your convenience—but be flexible. My Wednesdays every week were dedicated to cancer. The other six days were mine. I worked hard with the scheduling teams to keep appointments scheduled on Wednesdays, with exceptions when needed.

I chose to cold cap in order to minimize hair loss and that added complexity to infusion scheduling as not every infusion chair can be used. In partnership with the infusion center, I scheduled my infusions, directly, three months out, initially, and monthly thereafter. It was empowering! I could prioritize my treatments and coordinate my calendar with the center's availability. Taking this hands-on approach made the process smoother and helped me feel more in command.

Speaking of infusions—they're inevitable, so I chose to design my best infusion experience. After treatment, I learned a few things on which I could base my design. My infusion routine isn't unlike preparing for a long cross-country flight:

- Uniform – Fleece and comfy pants with a top made port access easy. Fluffy slippers kept feet comfy, except when using the ice socks to stave off neuropathy.

- Arrival – Get there early for port draw/labs. The sooner my labs came back, the sooner infusion started.

- Fill the downtime – Prepare a playlist, videos, or books to help you relax during the time between lab draw and pre-treatment, and if you wake up from your Benadryl nap.

- Environment – Eliminate the hospital antiseptic smell with an aromatherapy pendant, like lavender or bergamot.

- Coordinate the sequence of pre-treatment – I liked having the Benadryl last to kick off my nap. I also requested that my cold cap be "placed" by the team prior to Benadryl.

- Accept help – I loved my warmed blankets, saltines, and tea.

- Protect your nap – Figure out a way for the nurses to scan your id bracelet without waking you up. My husband gave me a stuffed stegosaurus after my port placement, which wore my bracelet next to me.

- Food – Make a lunch plan. My friends provided a lunch for each infusion, either packed in my cooler or to-go from a nearby restaurant. My infusions were five-and-a-half hours long due to cold-capping pre- and post-infusion periods.

After an infusion, I wanted to relax, so planned ahead for creature comforts. I chose where I wanted to sleep or rest and ensured other people in the house could respect my space. For post-surgery, I planned to be on the first floor of our home in a quiet bedroom that had black-out curtains. I borrowed a massage recliner from a friend to have something comfortable and easy to rise out of. I bought seatbelt pillows and a mastectomy robe with four inside pockets to contain the drains. Sharsheret sent me a mesh bag to hang around my neck while showering and another drain-holding belt when not showering. These anticipatory moves made me comfortable post-infusion and post-surgery.

Finally, I was a co-pilot, not a solo pilot. I learned to communicate regularly and openly with my medical team. Side effects, concerns, and questions that may arise—they want to know! They were my allies, and their expertise was invaluable in managing my experience.

4. **Invest in mental strength**

No one wishes for cancer, yet I found the gifts that accompany the journey are many. For me, this may have been easier because of my confidence that this cancer was not life-threatening. It's okay to slow down, to be overwhelmed and mad. Cancer messed up my sister's wedding! Cancer messed up my son's Bar Mitzvah! Cancer kept me from seeing my son's debut year of college baseball on campus! Cancer also reconnected me with old friends. Cancer brought me new friends. Cancer created a habit for my college kids to call me almost daily, connecting me to their emerging adult lives.

I strengthened my mental wellness during my breast cancer experience a number of ways. Before beginning my treatment, I identified a psycho-oncologist, Sadie, who could support me through this emotional rollercoaster with compassion, understanding, and years of expertise. Having someone to focus on my mental well-being played a crucial role in providing a sounding board just for me. For example, early on, my UCSF team needed my actual pathology slides from Peninsula Hospital to confirm my pathology and start treatment. There were difficulties acquiring the slides, despite my eagerness to get going and complete. My initial offer to help was rebuffed and a week later was welcomed. The night between the UCSF's request for my help and the morning when I could expedite my slides was very stressful for me. I was worried we would have to delay treatment. My psycho-oncologist was available via phone, text, after hours to share wisdom. She assured me there was nothing left to do because I had completed everything I could for that evening. So, I rested. Invaluable.

In addition to Sadie, I considered additional support systems. I assessed that support groups were not my preferred method for seeking solace; although, I enjoyed participating in the Facebook Peloton Breast Cancer Survivors private group to offer support and share what I knew.

Infusion centers try to be uplifting and comfortable, and during my chemotherapy sessions, I met a woman who shared my condition and treatment schedule—my chemo buddy. We established a bond that allowed us to offer comfort, strength, and encouragement during the arduous process. This connection became an invaluable support system for both of us. She's now a dear friend. We both achieved a Pathological Complete Response (PCR)!

Prior to being diagnosed, I had signed up for a mental fitness coaching program, Positive Intelligence, to consider adding it to my business. I decided to proceed with the program during the first seven weeks of chemotherapy, and it provided me with invaluable tools for managing the emotional turbulence, unforeseen challenges, and delays that are inherent to this journey. I learned to nurture my mental resilience, enhance my mental fitness, and increase my capacity to cope with adversity. I'm a fan!

For me, investing in my mental health was just as important as attending to my physical well-being—both are essential components of being an effective co-pilot of the breast cancer experience.

5. **Welcome people's help but set boundaries**

Embracing the support of loved ones was both empowering and comforting during my breast cancer journey. I welcomed help, but also established personal boundaries to maintain a sense of normalcy and protect my mental health. Personally, I don't like to feel dependent on people and I react negatively to pity, but I knew I needed help and wanted support. Helping people understand how to best help you is a gift to both you and them.

For those who wanted to bring food, it was helpful to share meal preferences, including dietary restrictions, allergies, or food dislikes. I linked to Sign-up Genius from my CaringBridge, and my BFF, Jessica, managed the site. In the Sign-up Genius, we specified the quantity of food needed and the frequency and asked people NOT to bring food if they weren't signed up on the meal train. This prevented waste.

Jessica also created a Sign-Up Genius for a smaller group of people who could be drivers to take me to appointments, treatments, or errands. My husband would have gladly done it all, but it's a lot and I wanted him to keep working and needed him to be there for me when it was impossible to schedule (like 2 a.m.). I wasn't allowed to drive home after chemo because of Benadryl, so I invited reliable and punctual friends to drive because time matters. It became a great way for me to catch up with friends. My chemo buddy drove herself to and from. It's a personal choice. When others drove me, I always had a backup driver in case of a problem (my sister was my backup).

I loved that people wanted to help and to see me, but it can get tiring. This is another opportunity to set some boundaries about preferences for visitation, including when and how frequently visitors should come. Once I learned that I slept through infusions, I let people know they didn't need to stay! I was honest with friends and family, explaining that I needed to recover and recharge, yet also welcomed supportive visits during periods of increased energy. My energy didn't dip a lot, but I became a lot more conservative about being in enclosed, indoor, and crowded spaces with a suppressed immune system.

My family is spread out, but wanted to help, so I asked specific tasks of loved ones based on their strengths. For example, my eldest (in college in Ohio) was my infusion-day DJ and created playlists for me, while my second son (in college in New York) wrote me heartfelt letters on infusion day as a special treat for me. My daughter, at home with me, was supportive and entertaining. My spouse, sister, college BFF, sisters-in-law, and parents were emotional pillars, while Jessica was the coordinator of practical support such as meals, driving, and visits. She was also my exercise buddy.

6. **Live your life and create moments to cherish**

Despite the challenges that come with a breast cancer diagnosis, embracing life and living it to the fullest feels even more important. Treatments may be demanding on body and mind, but finding joy in everyday activities helped me maintain my mental, emotional, and physical well-being. Life, even with cancer, is a gift and every day is a blessing, even if it's a hard day.

Because I was hands-on with my treatment schedule and communicating with my medical team, I was able to travel from California to Florida and upstate New York during my treatment to watch my freshman son play baseball, visit with my parents, and celebrate my twenty-fifth anniversary. These experiences provided a much-needed escape and the opportunity to create lasting memories. Just be back on Wednesdays!

I stayed involved in my children's activities, like attending their soccer and lacrosse games, which provided entertainment, normalcy, and mutual happiness. I wrapped myself in a warm coat and blanket to watch my daughter play, to cheer her on, and enjoy the fresh, crisp outdoor air.

I elected to cold cap my head during infusions. Cold capping is a non-invasive technique that can help protect hair follicles by reducing the scalp's temperature during chemotherapy, which decreases the amount of chemo that reaches hair cells. I was able to retain most of my salt and pepper mane. I had proactively bought a lovely hat collection and my sister-in-law sent me her wigs, but I never needed any of them. I didn't look like a cancer patient when I was out and about, which was excellent for my mental health and self-image.

Physical activity provided considerable benefits during my breast cancer journey. For me, weightlifting, metabolic conditioning, and walking helped maintain my energy levels and overall health amid the treatments. My BFF and I had been working out together for fourteen-plus years this way. During this time, she joined me in my home gym three days a week and we walked together one to two additional days. My doctors were amazed by my weekly laboratory results and the accelerated surgical recovery from the bilateral mastectomy and immediate DIEP flap reconstruction (needing no narcotics, walking the next day with a walker, healing in the top one percent of their experience). My body was primed to fast recovery because that's what happens in my workouts. It really helped.

Consult your healthcare team for guidance on suitable exercises for you. To minimize the impact of cancer on your health, embrace early detection and stay as strong and healthy as you can throughout your life.

Additionally, work was therapeutic for me. I enjoy achievement and connecting with people. Problem-solving creates energy for me. While I didn't work as much during treatment as I normally do, I continued working, learning, and teaching, since the focus on something other than cancer, connection to routine, and engagement were uplifting. Setting boundaries on the amount of stress and times available to work is crucial. If possible, request the flexibility you require.

While sex and intimacy may be different during the breast cancer journey, it remains an essential aspect of our emotional well-being. Due to the presence of chemotherapy drugs in bodily fluids, it's crucial to take your doctor's advice. It was awkward at times, but I didn't shy away from seeking pleasure and maintaining an intimate connection with my husband. I had to communicate my needs, desires, and fears and listen to his, but it built a stronger and more compassionate partnership.

By embracing life's moments and maintaining a semblance of normalcy amid the chaos, I reinforced my ability to cope with breast cancer and future crises. I listened to my body, set boundaries, and cherished the experiences and people that brighten my days.

Remember, we are more than our diagnosis. I am the co-pilot and a survivor, determined to live life on my terms.

Ludivine M.

The energy of saying Yes

Ludivine didn't wish to write an entire chapter, although she was determined to give voice to her soul. That's why she entrusted me with transcribing the content of our exchanges, which I am diligently striving to do as faithfully as possible. She thanks you, thanks you for taking the time to read, thanks you for pausing for a moment in a world where everything moves very quickly, where one must hurry to get sick, hurry to understand, hurry to heal, hurry to ...

Today, Ludivine is doing very well. She has found her path and her voice, she has healed from the pressures of performance, from most of her fears, and she walks her existence with confidence, with more joy and inner freedom. She sends her supportive smile to all those affected by cancer, and she sends a rose to all the authors of this book. She knows that we are all connected, beyond words and distances. I also thank her from the bottom of my heart for saying yes to life, and yes to this book. It has been an honor and a grace. Merci.[4]

Sophie Roumeas on the behalf of Ludivine M.

----

[4] Merci in French means « Thank you » in English.

Ludivine M.
The energy of saying Yes

*The real voyage of discovery consists
not in seeking new landscapes
but in having new eyes.*
–Marcel Proust

She advanced without saying a word, with her frustrations, fears, shortcomings, and difficulties.

Only she knew what her mind was telling her. The shame of not being able to change her aspirations, having to tell everything to those who didn't listen and nothing to those who should have.

Without knowing how to break free from this cycle, she sank into denial of her own power, until darkness took hold of her hands. Imprisoned in this irrational fear of being nothing, her divine mirror shattered, she stopped along the way, barely having time to realize what she had broken. Was it the cancer that served as her excuse, or was it the excuse that used the cancer? Who was this excuse?

Not content with being unable to dissolve the veil between the outer reality and her inner reality, the tone of life escalated, and soon a violent wind tore through the silence of her mismatched nights. No. No to violence, no to fading life, no to frustrations, no to everything that hurt her. Gradually, the energy of Yes diminished, and the sound of her voice became muffled by the noises of daily life.

She didn't have any more fear than reason; she simply didn't know. Nor did she understand what prevented her from appreciating the love of her man. What stood between her and the light of happiness was called shyness, anxiety, remnants of a past that had seared the valleys of her heart.

Aware that her emotions were preventing her from moving forward, she turned to the light of mutual assistance. She discovered that she was in no way solely responsible for this state of fact. Thus, the inner voice of truth began to awaken and heal its dormant and wounded octaves.

What to do with my emotions? What to become when the body has been invaded by an intruder? The myriad feelings of invasion-related turmoil connected with cellular predation ...

The voice whispered to her, "Learn to write your wounds in the sand and etch your joys in stone."

Finally, everything changed, remarkably. The noise of the wounds diminished until it became the gentle breeze's breath and the music calling for introspection.

*****

"I walked that path too ..."

It has been twenty years now since she embarked on the journey of becoming her own muse. Not far from that decision, the shadow of perdition kept her awake, never to fall asleep again.

In a society where it is fashionable to know how to fade away in favor of others, the paradigm shift of a highly sensitive person with a tumultuous childhood is not a straight path. Rather, it's a journey through the mountains, with turns on the sunny slopes and descents into the valleys of soul wounds.

> *Your daily life is your temple*
> *and your religion.*
> *–Kahlil Gibran*

When Ludivine receives her diagnosis, the whole world seems to have changed. What was important to her yesterday suddenly appears superfluous, and the superfluous from the day before, namely taking care of herself, suddenly becomes important.

"But how did I get to this point?"

That evening, when she felt a cyst in her right breast, already seems so distant. And yet, it's only been seven days. Seven short days that could have been ordinary have become as profound as what God must have felt when creating the world and humanity.

Day One: the creation of light (the diagnosis) ... on a reality that had remained invisible to her. Yes, she had been tired for months, maybe even years, but hadn't she been taught not to complain or listen to herself? The diagnosis confirmed what she had refused to feel; exhaustion as the illness progressed within her.

Day Two: the division of the waters, the sky, and the earth ... yes, her body had become independent from her mind and even her spirit. In reality, this step had taken her some thirty-five years of family responsibilities, career, and social life. Make no mistake. Not all lives undergo the same division as the one that had robbed her cells of the detection of the unwelcome host.

Day Three: the gathering of waters, the emergence of land and plants, life. After the shock of the past diagnosis, everything precious to her comes back to mind, even more precious than before. Her children, her husband, her friends, her family, her cat, her projects ... gathering inner waters with the battered body and thoughts of hope.

Day Four: organizing space, Earth, Sun, Moon ... Yes, she could no longer allow the victim part of her past to dictate her reactions to the whims and storms of destiny; it was time for her creative femininity to join forces with the strength of her original character to meet the needs of healing and anchor into life.

Day Five: the creation of the animal kingdom; when instincts had been suppressed to the point of confusing social conformity with personal aspiration, it was high time to rekindle intuition and the wisdom that precedes it.

Day Six: the creation of Man. The number six represents the soul. When had she managed to disable the inner elevator that allowed her to access the floor of her soul?

Day Seven: the day of rest, of completeness. A word whose meaning she had forbidden herself since the death of her young brother, a decade ago; some tragic events, despite urging one towards the path of acceptance, do not exclude the responsibility they entail towards those who remain.

Day Seven, today, the day of writing, of unleashing the un-childlike and outwitted speech. Ludivine contacted me in 2016 for the first time, after an event that could have cost her youngest son's life. That summer had brought together her greatest fears, thwarted her professional plans, touched her deepest values, and sowed doubt in her mind.

When Ludivine finally decided to make room for self-expression, our first work was on doubt. Doubt that opposed trust. What did she need to trust life again? At first, she didn't really know. Then, a few months later, she wrote these words, accompanied by a portrait photo of herself, with her hair cut and a determined sparkle in her eyes. She had found her answer, and she was now cherishing it dearly: "Rediscovering the path of the sacred, and the sacred begins within me."

*****

I pray because I believe there is something inside of me—and inside of every other human being that is holy and that the holiness in me is connected to the holy in everything else.
—Margie Klein

In addition, here is an excerpt of wisdom distilled by Father Étienne de Mesmay, honorary canon of Notre-Dame de Paris, regarding doubt and faith, that we used to read together with Ludivine:

"Is doubt the enemy of faith?

Faith in God is placing my trust in someone's word because they tell me they love me, and I dare to believe it's true. Doubt is when, from time to time, I question things. Does He really love me? It's the same in marital life: "I love you, and you, do you love me?" Doubt is a part of this relationship, which is a living relationship, in an area where no measuring instrument exists. Therefore, we will progress in this way, by asking questions, by evolving; we will take root, and we will arrive at a deep relationship of trust and love. In truth. Doubt is a part of faith. Conversely, if instead of doubt, you introduce suspicion, you are deliberately oriented toward something. You will have to find the flaw. Suspicion always leads to mistrust. Trust versus mistrust. With mistrust, the other can say almost anything to you, and you will always misinterpret what they say. You have severed the connection; you can no longer welcome acts of love or expressions of sympathy ... everything they say is false. You are completely isolated, separated; you can no longer communicate; you can no longer receive anything. It's like cutting off the connection with the Lord.[5] Faith is the current that flows; it is trust. And only trust can lead you to love."

> *At the bottom of great doubt*
> *lies great awakening.*
> *–Hakuin Ekaku*

---

[5] With the divine, the sacred part of life ...

Magali Rochereau
A glimmer becomes light

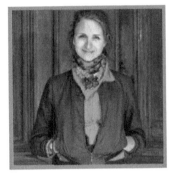

Magali Rochereau is forty-seven years old, with a husband, Philippe, and three sons, Jack, Louis, and Michel.

Magali has always been a Parisian and worked as a physiotherapist and osteopath until 2017 when she was diagnosed with breast cancer.

The upheaval of the illness made her reconsider the professional angle of her life, which represented a large part of time. She allowed herself to shake up everything she had built up until then, to pursue her dream of radio, music, and voice.

She currently works at the microphone of France Inter and Fip, to her greatest delight.

Instagram: @acoupdepour.quoipodcast

Facebook: magali rochereau

Linkedin: magali rochereau

Podcast: https://podcast.ausha.co/magali-rochereau

Magali Rochereau
A glimmer becomes light

One day at a time.

I feel like I've always lived in anticipation, in every sense of the word. I anticipated everything so as not to be caught off guard. I was never in the present moment, always waiting for something to happen. It couldn't just be "this." Yet, I was well off, a Parisian, at the helm of my private physiotherapy practice, with wonderful children and a loving husband. But I was waiting for something else. My days were repetitive and seemed like mountains of boredom to climb with bare hands. My mornings were discouraged before even opening my eyes.

And everything changed.

The story begins in the fourth month of my third son's pregnancy, one afternoon while I'm working in my office in Paris near the Arc de Triomphe. Seated at my desk between two patients, in front of my computer, my right-hand rested on my left breast, I felt a large lump under my fingers.

Fear. And yet, I do nothing with this information. I place it in a far corner of my consciousness and continue my work until July 31st, the date of my vacation and maternity leave. That day, among all the patients passing through my hands, I receive a particularly difficult lady who pushes me to my limits, like I've rarely been in almost twenty years of caregiving. I wonder about the meaning of this trial on this last day of work.

I don't know that day, but I will never return to work in my clinic.

My son is born in October. As I undress at the Les Halles pool, where I go whenever I have a few minutes to swim, I see that my breasts are entirely asymmetrical from each other, despite never having nursed any of my children and my body having regained its shape after childbirth. The right breast is rather flabby and saggy, while the left breast is extremely high, toned, and beautiful, as if it's housing an implant. I don't worry about it, but my friend Virginie, a gynecologist, takes the information very seriously and arranges a mammogram as soon as we talk on the phone. I'm standing on a street in my neighborhood at this very moment. I stop, looking at the sidewalk. I feel an alarm inside me go off.

Diagnosing this hormone-dependent Stage 3 breast cancer will be very laborious. It's an infiltrating carcinoma, and it's invisible. It's eventually discovered through a blind biopsy. Indeed, it takes up all the space in my breast. The doctor can't miss it. When the news comes, I'm at Virginie's clinic, and she tells me, "I don't have good news."

And in all simplicity, in a single consultation, I'm catapulted into the world of the sick. There are the healthy, those who go about their business, who run after their bus, who think about their dinner; those who have problems at work. And then there's me who has cancer.

I ride my motorcycle through beautiful Paris to go home and tell Philippe, who shares my life. I'm late. I didn't call. He knows where I was. Eyes filled with reproach. He would have wanted reassurance sooner because he doesn't believe in this disease story.

"It's cancer."

We have to stop. We have to sit down and listen to what the doctor friend has to say. Life will change. Maybe later you'll have to find meaning.

To save my life, the mission falls on the Curie Institute. I step into this parallel world, sobbing. The first visit is reassuring, the surgeon is optimistic. "We need to operate urgently, madam. It's taking over the whole breast. We won't hesitate. We'll remove the left breast in fifteen days."

And then the escalation of scans: PET scans, ECGs, MRIs, blood tests. Let's quickly find out everything; let's quickly understand everything to better encircle this dark beast that's eating away at me.

A wonderful piece of news can be hidden within a vile nightmare: the cancer is localized in the breast.

The moment is chosen to talk to the children just before the Christmas holidays, these holidays including a hospitalization for breast removal surgery between the two celebrations. We explain to them that I have been diagnosed with cancer during a breakfast picnic on the parental bed before heading to school.

It's Christmas, then my birthday. This year, my forty-third year, its shadow stretching before me and during which I am condemned to confront. Let's face it. I still have no idea what awaits me. Leaving early in the morning to remove a breast, leaving early in the morning to remove a cancer.

The surgeon sticks his head under the curtains before the operating room, "I found suspicious cells in the lymph nodes, I'm removing the whole chain."

Alarm!

Then it's a flat life on the left side. I fill my bra. I disguise myself. I conform. It doesn't occur to me that I could be different, be myself.

I recover from my surgery until the day of the results, of the analysis of the amputated breast. "It's a 12cm tumor and 12 lymph nodes are affected by cancer. It's serious and massive. In some cases like yours, some people have survived."

Stupor.

Stupor.

Stupor.

How do you activate your resources when your back is against the wall? Where do you find the strength to stand up? How do you manage to get up and fight? What should we believe in? I search for hope. Where is hope please? These questions obsess me. They will never leave me. Soon I will change my profession and create a podcast to help those in difficulty and to relish in the answers of others.

Months of degrading treatments during which I learn, day by day, who this woman in the mirror is. Isn't it crazy to start getting interested in her after forty-two years of cohabitation? What becomes interesting? What's at play? What becomes glaringly obvious in this great vulnerability? It's me who becomes glaringly obvious, me completely naked, me without artifice, me with all my fragility, me with my colossal strength. And that's new and beautiful. A self of love.

"I want to live."

After all the chemotherapy treatments, we decide to go beyond the helpless gaze of my doctors. *Andiamo* to Italy, as a family, camping or staying at an *agriturismo*. We'll laugh. We'll eat truffles. And we'll drink spritz. And I'll come back with a new tumor in the other breast, invisible on examination in France. You can be happy and smile while living an impossible situation. Fear always.

Upon my return to Paris, I ask to have that breast removed. I want to live. It's agreed.

The following year gives me back my hair, then soon my breast with the help of reconstruction, and life restarts and I return. How smiling is this journey back to normalcy that composes us, without false ideas of femininity norms.

Slowly, inexorably, a new path opens before me, little by little I allow myself to question the work that composes my life. Slowly, I give myself a chance, and more.

This renewal first takes the form of professional guidance, then a skills assessment, and sometimes a few seconds of magic opens a door and I rush into it like a voice into the mesh of a microphone: a radio training, a temporary job far from home, hold on, a calm time, a phone call. And it shifts. An exciting temporary job in Paris, a calm time, an announcement for an internship at the dream place. And it shifts again. The recruitment for the fairy's job.

A rain of stars and Walt Disney.

It would be misleading to think that's all. That we turn hell into paradise. That life accepts revenge. It would be misleading to create the word "resilience" and be content with it.

At the moment, I step into the long-awaited universe. A comfort ovary removal incidentally teaches me that cancerous cells from my breast have been detected in this new organ. Metastatic cancer.

I must do an extension search to find out if I am invaded by metastases. These moments, with their malignant strength, are very intimate, and they infinitely teach us about ourselves and about the meaning we give to the time allotted to us, to our destiny. I am alone. We are alone at the wheel of our life.

PET scan, terror, solitude, and faith. When the stakes are too immense and the terror too overwhelming, faith arrives. It can take various forms depending on each of our beliefs, but it is necessary for us to have a sacred place to gather, to lay down arms, to rely on something higher. "Your PET scan is perfect."

Infinite joy.

Here I am today in a situation where I am closely monitored by the medical field, which gives me targeted therapy to protect me. My challenge is to accept being at risk. Through EMDR (Eye Movement Desensitization Reprocessing), I manage to place the two traumatic cancer announcements in the past of my brain, to rejoice in accessing the job I've dreamed of my whole life, to smile at those hours of luck that I spend surrounded by my loved ones, because ultimately life is a high-risk journey for all of us.

Isn't it?

Philippe Andreani
Metanoïa

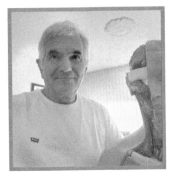

Osteopath DO, member of the French Register of Osteopaths.

President of the Ginkgo Biloba Health and Wellness Association, Medical and Paramedical Practice with Sophie Rouméas and seven French therapists, 24 Henri Bordeaux Street, 74000 Annecy, France.

Director of Research in Infrared Thermography, consultant for FLIR, particularly for breast cancer screening.

Dr Andreani work as an author and speaker:

Creator of the IPPAAR experience (Information, Physiological Preparation, and Anatomical Repair Area).

Webmaster of the website www.conquetedufroidinterieur.com, translated into English by FLIR

Two books: *Anatomy of a False Movement*, which now illustrates Physics and Chemistry textbooks for final year classes; available in French on Amazon: *Anatomie d'un Faux Mouvement*; and *False Movement Alphabet and Metanoia: Secrets of Anatomy*, available in French on Amazon as *Alphabet du faux-mouvement et Métanoïa*, published by BOD.

Infrared thermography illustration for the Health field in the Physics Chemistry textbook for final year science classes STI2D STL.

Published in osteopathic scientific journals: *Mains libres*, Switzerland, and *La Revue de l'Ostéopathie*, France.

Conference speaker at international osteopathy symposiums in Paris, France, Milan, Italy...

Email: phi.andreaniosteo@orange.fr

My work involves teaching Anatomy, and Anatomy is complex before it becomes simple. Therefore, I have endeavored to convey a simple, concise, and comprehensible anatomical message that makes sense to all and leads to greater awareness. It is sometimes amusing, but always in service of precise medical information.

Philippe Andreani
Metanoïa

Humans want to save the planet,
but what if the solution were simply
called "Anatomy"? It alone would be
capable of provoking the consciousness
upheaval known as "Metanoia.
—Andreani

To understand disease, we must explain what good health is. In this chapter, I will refer to French words, a frank speech between osteopath and patient, which helps to elucidate certain mysteries of metanoia.

*****

ANDREANI: You, me, everyone, to be well and to repair, to heal, to cicatrize, and even to prevent, we need oxygen, food, balance, muscles, nerves, tendons, rest, activity ... all the anatomical conditions must be met. We have several ways to hurt ourselves: either we fall off the bike, it bruises, or it's the weight of gravity, it causes osteoarthritis, the weight of years, the weight of kilos, the weight of worries, family, muddles, generations, legacies, viruses ... the weight of what you want.

What is certain is that we all receive a lot of information; thousands of pieces of information from morning until evening and even at night ... a bag of information. Some is pleasant and makes us happy and we do well. Others are stressful. It's getting on my ...

PATIENT: Nerves.

ANDREANI: I've got ... something in my throat ...

PATIENT: Yes, a lump.

ANDREANI: It hurts the stomach, hurts the back, hurts the head, hurts the knee, hurts the neck, hurts the breasts, hurts everywhere. And between the bag and us there is an arrow: information comes at us. How do we capture this information?

PATIENT: It's what we see on TV, what we read on Instagram, Whatsapp, what we hear on radio and what we discuss .... and what we feel.

ANDREANI: Is that how we learn about information: vision, audition, and sensation?

PATIENT: Absolutely.

ANDREANI: We could stop there, but your body would not be very happy. Because your body speaks to your brain and it says: First, I adore you. It's not complicated. I a-do-re you. We started together and we will end together, as long as things go well between us. But something saddens me, says the body to the brain. There's another way to capture information, but you're not talking about it. It's as if I counted for ...

PATIENT: Peanut butter.

ANDREANI: You know the French expression! Yes, it means „I'm useless at all." The problem is that I don't like counting for peanuts, and I'm going to send you a few messages, not very nice, moreover, just so that you remember me, don't blame me. I like you a lot, but this is you who is kicking me out, so it's just to draw your attention to me, says the body to the brain.

Another way of capturing information?

PATIENT: The brain.

ANDREANI: The brain analyzes the information, but it is not the one that captures it.

PATIENT: Emotions.

ANDREANI: Emotions are born after we've read information.

PATIENT: ... I don't see.

ANDREANI: In fact, there is still another way to become aware of information, and you don't talk about it either. What are you thinking about?

PATIENT: Listen to each other.

ANDREANI: Certainly, but you've already said it, "To Listen." That's two kilos of peanut butter, that's a lot of peanut butter. We can't tell you it's going well; we'll tell you it's not, and we'll do it our way.

What if I told you that there is yet another way of capturing information and you still don't mention it ... because that's three kilos of peanut butter, you might as well open a creamery.

PATIENT: I really don't see.

ANDREANI: One concerns your muscles, your nerves, your tendons, the skin informs you from bottom to top; it protects against the shocks of microbes, from the cold, from the heat; it provides information on the atmospheric pressure, the caress, the care, we breathe thanks to it, we sweat through it ...

PATIENT: The skin ... the touch!

ANDREANI: Of course. Touch. It can't tell you it's okay, it'll tell you it's not. It might even send you a few little lumps ... nodules ... to tell you that it's not right. It would prove the importance that your body places on this, value that you have set aside. So vision, listening, touch. Does that remind you of anything?

PATIENT: Yes, the senses.

ANDREANI: These are the senses that capture the information. The brain does not capture anything. The brain analyzes the information. It puts it in memory and it sends feelings, emotions, reactions, and behaviors to the body. We call it the „feeling" and we work from it. That's why we say, „You can trust me because I go by feel." But before you sense, first you have to feel it. If you don't feel, you can't express what you sense. Emotion comes from the Latin *movere*, which means to get out of there. Even as it was Shrek who said it with the donkey: It's better when you're ...

PATIENT: Out!

ANDREANI: Finally, someone who knows Shrek.

How many levels of feeling do you have? Apparently two: vision, audition. And I helped you to remember touch. But we say it's the five ...

PATIENT: Senses.

ANDREANI: Two more are missing.

PATIENT: The smell!

ANDREANI: Of course, the smell, the sense of olfaction. „O" for oxygen. You will only have smell if you inhale. Olfaction is, therefore, inhalation, breath, flair. Without oxygen, no life. In a minute without it, you're dead. By not considering the sense of olfaction as necessary, it is as if the oxygen could no longer enter. The carbon dioxide can, therefore, no longer come out. It saturates your tissues with lactic acid ... „It does not circulate in my home, it causes blood pressure, cramps everywhere"...

There is still a sense lacking. What is the fifth sense?

PATIENT: !! Vision, smell, touch, audition ... What is the fifth!? I don't remember anymore. No. But wait ... it's unbelievable ... I have a memory lapse!

ANDREANI: Symbolically, it represents desire to do, to be, like in French *avoir envie*, to want or desire, *and en-vie*, in English you translate literally by a-live. It's important. Write it as you want. A-live.

Quebecers can help. They don't say, „I want to ride a bike, but I have **bleep** to ride a bike."

PATIENT: The need.

ANDREANI: It's not that. When your child tells you „It's not good to eat," you answer him, „Before you say you don't like it, just **bleep** it ... „

PATIENT: „...just taste it. „ The taste!

ANDREANI: You forgot the taste. „I have the taste to ride," say the people of Quebec. You're not lucky. It's the most susceptible of all the senses from a neurological point of view. It hates being neglected; it will make you pay dearly for your lack of consideration towards it. The simple fact of not mentioning it indicates feeling down; the fact of forgetting it is a sign of depression. And nine out of ten people don't mention it. The world is going very bad.

At the level of the skull, there are nerves. The cranial nerves: twelve on the right, twelve on the left. One for olfaction, two for audition, four for vision, five for taste, including the Vagus nerve. Its dysfunctions and pathologies alone fill nine of ten hospitals: pulmonary, cardiology, digestive, diabetes, depression, autoimmune disease ...

We are about memory: twenty percent per sense; you have forty percent of active memory left ... with a memory hole.

Do you still have taste when you eat?

PATIENT: Yes, however, it seemed I have less and yet I am very gourmand.

ANDREANI: These are the most sensitive people who put themselves aside. „If I start expressing my desires, it will cause havoc everywhere." You have set aside touch, olfaction, and taste. You are not the only one: Six out of ten people name only vision and audition. Appearance. We were formatted like this: the money, the look, the appearance. Only one out of ten people are able to identify sensors as senses and name them all the way through without forgetting a single one. Most of them are children.

Picasso said, „With your world of appearance you have lost the domain of the child: wonder." He's not wrong. Do you know a lot of people full of wonder around you?

PATIENT: No indeed.

ANDREANI: Angry people: nine out of ten. We did a philosophy lesson that lasted three seconds: the conscious and the unconscious. Here is the conscious: vision, audition. Here is the unconscious: touch, olfaction, taste. It is about making conscious what is unconscious. Too much pressure in vision damages the eyes. Too much pressure in audition damages the ear: vertigo, tinnitus. They all break my ears. Not enough consideration for touch, smell, and taste.

The body does not like too much or not enough. In both cases it is the wrong movement. The whole of the senses is called „**instinct**": Here is what you are left with. In an animal world with three less senses: run fast, a crocodile will soon eat you. Instinct is absolutely not an end. It's just a neuro-logical strategy to set up the basis for all repair, healing, and immunity. It's not because you pick upon well that you are spared from stress or viruses, but you are protected. It's like in *Survivor*[6]: an immunity necklace.

When returning from vacation, on the highway, five motor-way tolls are open. You close three of them, it's going to yell. I wouldn't like to be in your place at the toll on the highway.

„Do you open your tolls?"

„I lost the keys!"

The pressure rises in the open tolls: headlight calls ... which damage the view: glaucoma ... horn concert ... which damages the ear: tinnitus, vertigo. They all break my ears.

Two other tolls are opening quickly. One is resisting: The unions are getting involved. Understand the surgeons: Do

---

[6] *Survivor* is a popular reality television show that originated in the United States and has been adapted in many countries around the world. The show was created by Charlie Parsons and premiered in the U.S. in 2000. It is known for its unique format, competitive challenges, social dynamics, and strategic gameplay. In *Survivor*, a group of contestants are placed in a remote location and are divided into tribes. They must work together to provide food, shelter, and other necessities, while also competing in phys-ical and mental challenges to win rewards and immunity from elimination.

you want us to fiddle with the scalpel? Not very hot for that ... so open your toll! The circulation becomes fluid again: blood and nerve circulation.

You were instinctive and creative, you are not anymore, but you will return to it: Do you know how long it takes to get it back?

PATIENT: Not long I hope.

ANDREANI: Three seconds: time to remember the five senses, but without forgetting a single one ... taste, touch, smell, vision and ... audition. The magic of image: you can start creating, repairing, healing again. And your fifty-six billion cells aren't even resentful. It's true, we lost a bit of time ... but it was worth it. Look: What you had forgotten ends up at the head of the gondola, and vision and audition ultimately don't matter that much.

This reversal of the situation: What was forgotten becomes the priority, and what was quoted becomes less important. It has a name. It is called „metanoia": You have made a magnificent metanoia. I'll bet a million dollars you don't know what that means.

PATIENT: Exact.

ANDREANI: I'm willing to bet another million dollars you know „paranoia. „

PATIENT: Yes.

ANDREANI: Because we are in a world of paranoia. And I'll bet a third million dollars you don't know what „noia" means.

PATIENT: Exact.

ANDREANI: We don't know what it means, but we use it without problem to call others paranoid. „Noia" means consciousness, and „paranoia" means beside consciousness. We are nine out of ten to be beside ourselves, to be paranoid. Now you are in meta-noia: in consciousness and above: „I am the one who decides. I put them in the order I want," and then everything will change.

You will look in the metanoia dictionary: anatomical, neurological, psychological, and even spiritual reversal, a-live first. Remember the French, *en-vie*.

Does taste speak to you first and touch second?

PATIENT: Absolutely, I am very gourmand and everything touches me.

ANDREANI: It's always the most sensitive people who put themselves aside: *Ratatouille*[7] rising sign and very tactile. Now you are in a position to repair, heal, and also prevent. Above all, the awareness of our senses is the basis of all this cellular renewal. But instinct is absolutely not an end, it's just a step towards more awareness. The path is not over, but it's already a very good start to healing. In fact, this instinctual body is our real terrestrial vehicle: Where are the headlights of your car among the five senses?

PATIENT: Vision?

ANDREANI: Exact. Vehicle body?

PATIENT: Touch.

ANDREANI: Perfect. Balancing? It works with the horn, so that the car stays well on the road.

---

[7] The movie *Ratatouille* is the same in both France and the United States. It features the character Remy, a rat with a passion for cooking, who teams up with a young kitchen worker to create culinary masterpieces. *Ratatouille* is an animated film produced by Pixar Animation Studios and released by Walt Disney Pictures.

PATIENT: The ear, audition.

ANDREANI: Alright. Olfaction is oxygen, so it's the fuel for the vehicle, because without oxygen and without gasoline it doesn't move forward; and taste is to feel desire, a-live, remember *en-vie* in French, and desire is a hell of an engine.

That's an extraordinary car you've got there: Look at the engine size!

And the vehicle body is solid, plus it drives at night. It's ready for the 24 Hours of Daytona[8]. It's a Maseratti. You're driving a Maseratti! Did you know?

PATIENT: No, but I'm very happy to know it. It makes me happy. It gives me courage and energy.

ANDREANI: On the other hand, the previous car posed a problem. You dropped off two headlights and a horn at the garage for the technical control. The mechanic calls you back immediately. „I'm waiting for your car!?"

„But I dropped it off this morning!"

„Well, I can tell you that there will be no technical control."

„I'm delighted," you say.

„No! You can't be happy, because if there's no control, it's because there's no car!"

Now all your sensors are open, so you are an open person; before you were someone ...

PATIENT: Closed.

---

[8] The "24 Hours of Daytona," officially known as the "Rolex 24 at Daytona," is an annual endurance sports car race held at the Daytona International Speedway in Daytona Beach, Florida, USA. It is one of the most prestigious and well-known endurance races in the world.

ANDREANI: Now, let's return to the anatomy of French language: "open" in French means *ouvert*; and if you change the order of the letters from *ouvert*, another word will appear which will bring many solutions to your breast cancer challenge; anagram of *ouvert*?

PATIENT: Virtue ... *vérité* (*truth* in English) ...

ANDREANI: I'm sure you will find this is a quality of people who are open, and as per the sacred text, „Who seeks" ...

PATIENT: Will find!

ANDREANI: Yes, when you are open, you find, but closed, find does not work. However, let's return to the anatomy of French: *ouvert* rhymes with another, less sympathetic anagram: *voûter* in French „to vault." You are no longer curved as a vault; the V of vault representing the weight curving the back, from curved to cured, you can find the solution to this ordeal of cancer. A test at your level, and you will succeed. You are just ahead of seven billion people who'll have to make their own metanoia.

Someone once told me: It looks like a word from the future. It is, however, coming from the past. It is ancient Greek. There are many Greek and Latin words in anatomy, but it could become the word of the future. Anagram of metanoia? It could save Alzheimer's, the planet, and cancer. It is the universal language between all therapists in the world ... I wish you a beautiful journey and a beautiful anatomy[9].

And you, how do **you** get information?

---

[9] Anatomy is translated as *Anatomie* in French, the perfect anagram of Metanoia.

Sam Yau

A Medley of Poems selected from Sam Yau's poetry books *Soul's Journey* and *Souls in Love* co-authored with Sophie Rouméas

(Certain poems adapted for this anthology)

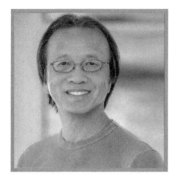

I have re-invented my life several times, from a six-month-old baby on a refugee boat to a penniless student from a distant land, to the CEO of a billion-dollar corporation, to the chairman of an iconic pioneering center for personal growth, to a poet who writes about the soul's journey, life's vicissitudes, trauma and healing, consciousness, and mysticism.

My poetic musings clarified, distilled, deepened, and ingrained the essence of past spiritual experiences onto my being. As I sculpted my poems, my poems sculpted me at the same time. Writing poetry has become my most enjoyable and uplifting spiritual practice.

I published my first poetry book, *Soul's Journey*, in 2021. I co-authored *Souls in Love* with my partner, Sophie Rouméas, in 2022. Both books became Amazon International Bestsellers.

I live with Sophie and my seventeen-year-old daughter, Sapphire, in Laguna Beach, California.

Website: samyaupoetry.com

Email: sam@samyaupoetry.com

Facebook: Sam Yau Poetry

Instagram: samyau_poetry

Sam Yau

A Medley of Poems selected from Sam Yau's poetry books *Soul's Journey* and *Souls in Love* co-authored with Sophie Rouméas

To heal is to return to love.
—Sam Yau

I am a soul

By Sam Yau

I am a soul
made in the image of God

I was never born
I will never die

Love will never end
for God is Love

I have no fear
for God is in me
I am in God

Light shall shine in my darkest days
I shall be filled with joy in my deepest sorrow

Gratitude

By Sam Yau

May the diagnosis be
a turning point

to expand rather than shrink
your life perspective

May your eyes be open
to witness the miracle
of being alive and grateful
for the simple pleasures
of daily living

Feel the cup of latte
warm your hands
let its delicate, sweet flavor
mellow your heart

Behind the barista
can you see the farmers
the processors, the distributors
from the four corners of the world
toiling to create this delight to start your day

How the window is eager to show you
the golden sunset over the Pacific
the stair tread to rise to receive
your next step as you ascend

the kettle to whistle
a tender love song
the oven to ooze the
the delicious aroma
of baking croissants

How the patient rocks grinded
against the ocean waves for eons
to turn into the finest white sands
to cuddle your feet on the beach

How floating moisture, dust, and wind
create the most gorgeous shape-
shifting clouds to dazzle you

How the Sun and the Moon take turns
to illuminate you from the sky
Can you see,
every encounter
is an exchange of love

How everything around you is alive,
forever saying, "I love you."

Gratitude unlocks
the hidden intimacy you
already have with everything

You have never been alone

Meditation
By Sam Yau

Thoughts fly into my mind's chamber
like uninvited birds
without attention from me
they can no longer latch
onto other thoughts
new arrivals become spare
One by one, they depart

Without thoughts
memories can't linger
tomorrow can't emerge
Without a flutter of past or future
my feelings subside

I WALKED THAT PATH TOO

Lying still, I feel
each pulsation in my wrist
the throbbing at my toes' tips
I hear the thundering rumbling
and growling in my guts
the whirling and gushing
of my arteries' blood
all sensations fall away
into quietude

With the last trace of breath gone,
my body vanishes

Floating in immense emptiness
submerging in cosmic silence
without any sense of self
losing all my boundaries
on the edge of the horizon
I disappear into a
vast awareness

Coming back
the quiet echoes
through my empty body

I have traversed the void
the fullest emptiness
I have ever glimpsed
shimmering with infinite
creative potential

My heart explodes

No longer am I a tiny speck
the universe is in me

Devour

By Sam Yau

Before morning peeks around the curtain's edge
before the memory of last night's dreams starts to fade
before I am hijacked by mental chatter
in the twilight between asleep and awake

I lie still
find my breath
sense my rhythm
tune in to what I'm feeling

in my body
without thinking
without judging

If the feeling has a color, I
let it seep across my entire field of vision
soak every cell of mine in its hue

Sometimes it is a golden lifting-up
other times, it is a gray heaviness in my chest
if I stay long enough with it
I reach its opposite

If the feeling has a taste, I
swish it around in my mouth
savor it with my electrified taste buds
some mornings are easier than others
but I don't try to cover it

I leave no trace of my hangover
I devour it
lick my palate clean
start fresh for a new day

Acceptance

By Sam Yau

My curriculum was designed
for my growth in this lifetime

May I have the courage
to embrace all experiences
as they unfold on my path

May I know I am here
to live my unique life

May I have the fortitude to
refrain from judging events
as good or bad

May I be wise enough
not to compare my realities
with those of others

May I step into my healing
by accepting what is

Accept, but don't succumb
to blame myself, so
I can discern what the
messenger has to say

In acceptance, I can fully
taste each unfolding and
feel and express my grief

May I be more intimate
with my soul to receive
clear inner guidance for
my healing journey

Return to Wholeness

By Sam Yau

Because of pain caused by trauma
you dissociate from your body

Because of never receiving enough love
you feel you're not good enough

Because of fear of disapproval
you hide parts of your being in the shadow

Because of a missing body part due to illness
you feel you're no longer complete

On the surface, you have lost so much of you

Brokenness
unspoken grief
emptiness

Yet everything you have lost or discarded
is still there in your energy field

Gather all of them
re-own and transcend them
for you have traveled far
from there, that is still yours
to here, where you live now

Soon, you will discover
your true nature
you are precious

totally lovable
complete and perfect

Come home to your body
the imperfections in your humanity
are still perfect in your divinity

Embrace the totality of your life's journey

Reclaim who you are

Discover the fullness
of being both divine and human

To heal
is to return to wholeness

The Nature of Love
By Sam Yau

Love binds
causes things
to come together
to interact

to co-create
to evolve
in an endless cycle of love

Love is the subtle vibration
that underlies the ocean of
interpenetrating fields
of energy and matter

Love is more fundamental than
electromagnetic, nuclear
and gravitational forces

Love invokes matter to become
life through alchemy

It is the mother of all feelings
it is the origin of all unions

Of life, love is
the sweetest nectar
the balm that heals
life's wounds and
its deepest longing

Its shadow is fear
fear of loss of love
fear of loneliness

The birth of all births
the creator of all creations
the thrust of all creative impulses

It is disguised as thousands of things
amid which we have forgotten our true essence

Love subdivides itself
into many forms of beauty

Beauty is in the eyes of the lover
the one who can no longer love
cannot see beauty in anything

Even truth is like a ray of light
that can be bent
in opposite directions
by the perspectives
of love
or fear

If you are a lover of all things
your stream of joy and bliss
is unceasing

You then live as your true being

You are love itself

Sandra Gropper

The elephant in the room

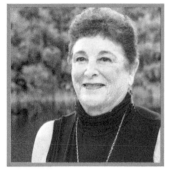

Sandra Gropper's roots trace back to Long Island, New York, in a small town beyond the rhythm of New York City. Her academic journey led her to Brooklyn College, a distinguished institution within the City University of New York, where she pursued a path in health and physical education.

Following graduation, Sandra embarked on a career as an educator. She imparted her expertise in physical education to students from seventh and eighth grades to high school. In addition, she shared her knowledge of health sciences with pupils in the sixth, seventh, and eighth grades.

During a pivotal phase of her life, Sandra dedicated a decade to nurturing her two daughters as a stay-at-home mother, eventually transitioning back to the professional realm, and making significant contributions to real estate where she engaged in data comparison at a real estate market research firm and worked in the office of a real estate developer.

Having been retired for thirty years, Sandra resides in the sun-kissed landscapes of southeast Florida, savoring the activities of her well-deserved retirement.

Sandra can be contacted at skgropper@gmail.com.

Sandra Gropper

The elephant in the room

Above all, be the heroine of
your life, not the victim.
—Nora Ephron

The date was November 5, 1983, when the elephant showed up. As I was taking a shower, getting ready for our Saturday night date with friends, I felt a small lump in my right breast. I asked my husband to come into the bathroom to see if he could feel the lump. He felt it. Said to myself, "Probably nothing." But as I was standing at the stove boiling pasta for my children's dinner, I became sure that it was something.

We told my sister-in-law. She contacted her doctor in New York City who referred me to Dr. Gene Nowak, a general surgeon. He fit us in for a late appointment on that following Friday, November 11. I don't remember getting a mammogram, but I must have. Cancer was confirmed ninety-nine percent.

Dr. Nowak spent over an hour with my husband and me discussing options. He recommended a unilateral mastectomy because I was young (thirty-six). Lumpectomies were relatively new, new enough that there wasn't more than five years of research on survival rates. Dr. Nowak wanted to go for a long-term survival. He explained what to expect of the reconstruction. At one point in our discussion, Dr. Nowak commented, "If you have a good marriage, this will make it stronger; if you don't have a good marriage, this will make it worse." We knew we had a strong marriage, a marriage that would certainly survive this forthcoming ordeal.

We called my parents after our meeting with Dr. Nowak. They flew in the next day, Saturday, the 12th. Surgery was scheduled for Monday, November 14, only nine days after I had discovered the lump, much sooner than procedures today.

We were so frightened. Not as much was known about breast cancer or any cancer then. All I kept thinking was that I wanted to survive to see my girls, Joelle and Tracey, grow up. I did a lot of crying that weekend.

At that time, I was a full-time health education teacher. I remember calling my principal to tell her what was happening. I told her that she would need to find a substitute for me because I didn't expect to return to work until after the New Year.

My husband drove me to New York Cornell Hospital on Sunday night. I guess in those days, if a patient stayed at home the night before surgery, they could not be trusted to abstain from eating or drinking after midnight.

As scheduled, on Monday, Dr. Nowak removed my right breast and many of the lymph nodes under that arm. Sentinel nodes were not known in 1983. I was in the hospital for eight days with several large drains the size of dinner plates. I couldn't go home until the drains were removed, which was approximately a week after surgery. While still in the hospital, I met with a plastic surgeon, Dr. Ken Rothhaus, who said I had to wait approximately six months before reconstruction could begin. Again, couldn't have been more different than today.

Amy was a special nurse at the hospital. She helped patients like me deal with the psychological ramifications of the surgery and met with me and my family. Amy was very kind and helpful, but that was all the support that was available at the time. In those days, people didn't talk about having cancer. Much less was known about cancer then. We feared that, if known, friends would withdraw socially, fearing that I was contagious. And when word did get out, we saw some people step away.

I came through the surgery and returned home. Radiation and chemotherapy were not required at that time. I thought I was done with the cancer, but it was like the elephant in the room. Even if I wasn't constantly thinking about it, the possibility of my cancer coming back someplace in my body was always present. Sometimes it was close, in my face, and sometimes it was in the corner. But it was always there!

I went on to have many reconstruction surgeries with implants which were done by Dr. Rothhaus, the plastic surgeon. The initial surgery involved placing a tissue expander (surgery one). Every other week, I had saline injected to expand the tissue expander. When the desired size was achieved, the expander was removed and a permanent silicone implant was put into the cavity (surgery two). This procedure was repeated two more times over the years due to implant ruptures, for a total of six implant surgeries. Lots of anesthesia and hospital stays put the elephant directly in my face.

I went back to teaching in January, but requested and was granted a part-time schedule, only four classes per day instead of my usual six, which school administrators accommodated. I was teaching a new health course in sex and drug education. Administrators were concerned that students' questions about sex and drugs would go beyond the district's brand-new curriculum and students' grade level. Such questions were not acceptable for me to answer and made me quite anxious. The new curriculum created additional challenges. For example, there were no supporting materials, so everything had to be created. There were no computers or printers in the school in 1983/84. The only duplicating method available was the labor-intensive, low-cost mimeograph, which squeezed ink through stencils, which I created and ran off myself.

In June after completing one semester post-surgery, part-time, I was asked to come back full time in the fall semester. I agreed but requested only two grade levels instead of the three that I had taught prior. Initially, the principal told me that that would not be a problem. However, in August she called to say that they could not accommodate my request after all. My husband and I were hesitant to agree because the previous year had created so much stress for me. Looking back, I should have asked for a schedule that included two or three physical education classes instead of all health. But I did not. So, I did not return to teaching that September.

About eighteen months after my initial surgery, I once again felt a small lump on the scar of the original surgery. I had already been scheduled to go into New York City to see Dr. Rothhaus, my plastic surgeon. Up until this point, my husband had taken me to every appointment in the city. But I thought that perhaps the lump had something to do with the implant, so this time I said, "I'm just going to the plastic surgeon for a checkup. You do not have to take me. I'll take the train."

Well, the lump had nothing to do with the implant. When Dr. Rothhaus, whose office was in the hospital, saw the lump he said, "Let's see what this is," and ushered me into his procedure room. I was given a local anesthetic and we joked around until he saw what it was—the cancer had come back. He left me with his nurse and called Dr. NowakNowak, my general surgeon, to get further instructions as to whether he should remove the whole tumor, how much of a margin he should take, and what he should tell me.

My poor husband, Malcolm. He was all the way down in Toms River, New Jersey, at a builders meeting—a one-and-a-half-hour drive to New York City without traffic. It was Passover and Dr. Rothaus was a practicing Jew whose family was waiting for him for the second seder. Malcolm arrived about seven o'clock, but until he did, Dr. Rothhaus and his nurse would not leave me.

Next, I scheduled an appointment with Dr. Nowak. He told me I would need chemotherapy and radiation. Chemo was very different then, though some of the drugs are still in use today. Dr. Nowak recommended Dr. Gene Resnick, an oncologist, who would prescribe and administer the chemotherapy. I had 5-FU (Whatever that is!), Methotrexate, Cytoxan, and Prednisone, the only anti-nausea medicine available at the time. The 5-FU was administered in Dr. Resnick's office with a slow injection into a vein. Probably one of the reasons why my veins aren't in good shape today. I took the Methotrexate and Cytoxan orally and continued this regimen for one year. The elephant was smacking me right in my face. After about three months, I took a break from chemo so that I could have five weeks of radiation. The radiation therapy was done locally.

While I was going through the first half of chemo, a friend and neighbor called to tell me about a doctor in New York, an endocrinologist/oncologist, who had done wonders for a friend of hers with a vitamin/mineral therapy. So, we made an appointment to see him. He prescribed a vitamin regimen for me which I followed. Couldn't hurt.

I had lost my hair from the chemo which was very traumatic. I remember standing in the shower crying as my hair came out in bunches. When we took a break from chemo for the radiation treatment, my hair started to grow in. When chemo was restarted, I did not lose my hair again. I can only attribute it to those vitamins. I still take many of the same vitamins today.

During this time, I began to see a psychiatrist, Dr. Martin Bier, to help me deal with my fears, the elephant in the room, and the chemotherapy. At one point, he suggested that I find an additional activity that I could enjoy, besides tennis, which I had continued to play two times a week through everything. I found a folk-dance group that met one night a week in Red Bank in a parking lot adjacent to the Navesink River. I joined the group until my wig was inadvertently knocked off one night. My partner was mortified, and I was foolishly embarrassed and never returned to the group again.

During this time too, I was very involved as neighborhood group leader for the Girl Scouts. During one of our meetings, a condolence card was distributed because a neighbor, the one who was doing so well on the vitamin regimen, had just died from breast cancer. It was her endocrinologist/oncologist that my husband and I had seen and the same protocol of vitamins I was following. I had a full panic attack. A friend got me out of the meeting, and we called my husband, who came home. I then called my general surgeon, Dr. NowakNowak, but heard from his partner, Dr. Clark. He was wonderful. We talked for about thirty minutes, and he calmed me down. I later learned that he was suffering from terminal cancer himself. An amazing man.

In 2013 my younger daughter, Tracey, at twenty-nine-years old and engaged to be married, was diagnosed with breast cancer. It was then that we found out that she was BRCA1 positive. I was tested and found to be positive for BRCA1 as well. I knew of no one else in my family who had had breast cancer.

I had a decision to make.

As BRCA1 positive, I stood an eighty-percent chance of another breast cancer and/or ovarian cancer. I decided to have a hysterectomy, as I was well beyond childbearing age. But I still had to decide if I would have another mastectomy.

Admittedly, I was never happy with my previous reconstructions, which I had pursued vigorously. Then sometime in 2014, my husband had a conversation with his cousin Jill, who had had a double mastectomy and a DIEP flap reconstruction, reconstruction that uses the woman's own tissue, at MD Anderson Medical Center. My husband insisted that we go and visit with Jill to learn more. She took me into the bedroom and showed me the results of her procedures. I was amazed. We took down the name of the doctor and I made an appointment with him.

Dr. Geoffrey Robb was a world-renowned plastic surgeon specializing in DIEP flap reconstruction. He indicated that I would be a good candidate for the procedure.

My decision was made. I would proceed with the second mastectomy and DIEP flap reconstruction. It was not an easy decision, but my life, my survival, was my primary concern. Given that I was BRCA1-positive, the chance of another cancer was too great. I was all in and immediately scheduled the surgery.

The DIEP flap surgery was successful, albeit our stay in Houston was extended due to a hurricane in Florida where we were living at the time. I am happy that I had the procedure.

While it may not be perfect, it certainly is an improvement. There would be no more reconstructive surgeries for me.

In January 2023, my oldest daughter, Joelle, who was also BRCA1 positive, was scheduled for prophylactic bi-lateral mastectomies with DIEP flap reconstruction. When my youngest daughter, Tracey, was diagnosed, I had panicked. But after living through my experience, I learned that cancer does not have to be a death sentence. So, when Joelle was diagnosed my response was different. I was much calmer and waited for the results of the biopsy and doctors' recommendations. Having been through the process three times before, once with Tracey and twice myself, I had learned several lessons: (1) stay calm (2) keep a positive attitude and relax as much as possible; (3) accept help and support from your friends, family, and community; (4) find the best doctor you can who is associated with a major hospital; and (5) trust your doctor and follow the protocol.

All my doctors were caring and wonderful. My family was there with me every step of the way. My husband and I recently celebrated fifty-five years of marriage with our entire family of two beautiful daughters, two sons-in-law, and five extraordinary grandchildren. I consider myself blessed and fortunate that I have been able to live a full and active life since diagnosed with cancer almost forty years ago.

Stephen and Cecile Baudin

A couple of therapists

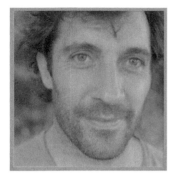

Stephen Baudin's therapeutic journey is far from being conventional; rather, it follows a dreamlike thread. Initially, he studied dreams, exploring their extensions and their connections to the waking world under the guidance of Roger Zanoni. This foundation laid the groundwork for his ongoing development, continuing in the company of Mr. Zanoni since 1992. His interest then turned to metaphysics, which he studied with two erudite former students of Maurice Guinguand.

Simultaneously, he delved into Taoist Chinese medicine with one of the pioneers of integrating biological decoding into acupuncture, Mr. René Zeender. In 2000, he graduated from the Zhao Bichen Institute as an acupuncturist. He opened his practice and then, in 2004, traveled to the Ladakh plateaus to study Amchi medicine with Chief Amchi Phumtsok. In Ladakh, he encountered a therma (hidden teaching by Padmasambhava) that he stabilized under the guidance of His Holiness Ogyen Trinlé Dorjé, the 17th Karmapa, on the 17th day. He entered a year-long meditation and, following the advice of His Holiness, began teaching this therma, swiftly intertwining it with his teachings on Chinese medicine.

Starting in 2010, he engaged in therapeutic follow-up with patients of Dr. Philippe Lagarde. The latter taught him the Heitan-Lagarde test for monitoring cancer rebound effects in patients. In 2013, he settled in Switzerland and founded the Ling Dao Center, which offers various courses, including a federal curriculum in Chinese medicine.

www.centrelingdao.ch

https://vitacomplex.shop

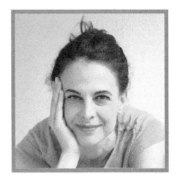

Cécile Taric-Baudin is a therapist and a yoga and meditation teacher. Transitioning from a professional dancer to a consultant in new technologies, it was an initiatory journey around the world with a backpack that transformed her perspective on existence and way of life. For over fifteen years, she wandered the globe seeking medicinal and spiritual teachings at their source, living with masters, healers, and yogis in countries such as Guatemala, Mexico, India, and Nepal. It was in Thailand that she began training in energetic medicines, then she followed the path of the Maya and studied shamanism in Central America under Don Lauro de la Cruz. The understanding of the Self through energy captivates her and leads her to specialize in secret Tibetan yogas.

She intensely practices the path of awakening, with years of solitary yoga retreats (including the Six Yogas of Naropa) and meditation guided by her Geshe Lobsang Choephel. From a young age, Cécile was convinced that the universe is energy and that the energetic power inherent in every being constitutes an unlimited source of healing.

Today, she shares her knowledge and supports those who suffer or seek to evolve in their self-understanding and inner motivations. In 2021, she opened her center in Switzerland, offering individual consultations while organizing workshops, retreats, and training in energy healing, yoga, and meditation.

www.ceciletaric.org

Stephen and Cecile Baudin

A couple of therapists

... These people walk only to seek resources,
and the source of dreams dries up.
—Gustave Kahn

My name is Stephen Baudin, and I have been a specialized therapist in oncology for many years. My story is not about my skills, nor my professional understanding of cancer, at least not directly. I will narrate the process that led me to encounter this disease and become a specialized therapist. This narrative does not have a personal objective, but rather aims to shed light on the subtle mechanisms that healing from cancer offers.

Each cancer encompasses a multitude of existential and hereditary data that I invite you to observe in the form of a loop. Only a loop allows making sense of a range of understandings, whether positive or negative, while also allowing for retracing one's steps and maintaining the same guiding thread. If we no longer perceive the full spectrum of colors and our view of the world narrows to black and white, we approach the feeling of a woman when she learns that her breast is affected. The color of her life fades abruptly, making way for apprehension about the long therapeutic process that quickly emerges. This black-and-white view is nothing but a skillful blend of shadow and light. This so-called autoimmune disease signifies the transformation process of our light into shadow—cancer. This binary perspective reveals that healing requires reversing this now-biological process, not through relentless positivity, but through a clarity inherent in the mechanism of the loop.

Armed with my studies in Chinese medicine, with a sense of easily directing energy, I intertwine this knowledge with the biological decoding of the 1990s. Like a freshly graduated psychologist, I believe I know before I see. I had reached the pinnacle of therapeutic presumption, aiming to gain power over the patient's psyche. As with any premature ascent, I needed to discover, internally, the reasons behind this egotistical expansion. Like a hero following the footsteps of ancient Greece, I journey to the Himalayas and Tibetan medicine. Along the path of learning this medicine, I stumble upon a small pebble that generates grand dreams within me. My quest continues until I meet His Holiness the Karmapa, to illuminate these dreams that my consciousness had held onto as the gears of a grand design. As a spiritual father, His Holiness highlights the precious nature of the teachings hidden within this pebble by the Tibetan Buddha. But the question is, "What do you want to do with them?"

I was perplexed. I had thought this meeting would provide some sort of guidance, but now I had to give direction to these dreams myself. "I would like to teach them," I instinctively reply.

"In that case, you will need to stabilize these teachings," retorts His Holiness.

I was at the height of my spirits, my mind bathed in the nectar of a treasure. As I left His Holiness and descended the stairs, accompanied by two armed soldiers, the realization struck me. "What does it mean to stabilize a teaching?" Suddenly, I became aware that my initial intention in this entire journey is not healthy. I am doing all this to gain my own biological father's recognition. And having been a competitor in my youth, I know that an intention not rooted in a healthy foundation sooner or later leads to an accident.

One morning, Roxane, a longtime friend, called me. She informed me about her breast cancer that had spread to her ovaries and was in the process of invading her peritoneum. Unbeknownst to me, I developed a multitude of therapeutic techniques alongside her aimed at drying out her cancerous foci. And it worked. This caught the attention of the oncology professor who was treating Roxane, and he asked me to come and meet at his clinic. Quickly, I began taking care of a significant portion of his patients. At that moment, I realized that the teachings I had discovered in the Himalayas were directly related to cancer. Unfortunately, Roxane left us after many years of respite. I continued to accompany another patient of the professor, Valérie, who had become a friend through numerous clinic encounters. Following Roxane's passing, I needed to find a balance between the warmth of the trust bond and the coldness of the resolution of this disease. This cannot be learned. It imposes itself on our receptivity, in a strange way over time. This balance then allowed me to explore the relevance of cancer cells, which are both informed by the patient's life history and entirely autonomous in exploiting their host's body. My fascination with the intelligence of the disease gradually led me to understand it, to sense whether it is magnanimous or unleashed, such as when it mutates. But let's return to our loop of understanding.

This disease is confrontational; it imposes itself upon the patient, especially when the weight of therapeutic measures begins to take effect in their life. I often hear questions like, "What's happening?" or "Why aren't the results matching my suffering?" A friend confided that on her deathbed, accepting her end, when everything was ready for her departure, she woke up after sensing the veil of her cancer had lifted. "I saw my life unfold and accepted its outcome," she told me. The ways of fate are inscrutable, but in this particular case, accepting the intricacies of the disease allowed her to live. She has now been free of relapses for thirty years. Indeed, the cancer must not return. From experience, the rebound effect, the recurrence of cancer, depends on this loop of understanding. However, how can the patient identify their own loop? This remains mysterious and requires humility from the therapist.

There are as many therapeutic approaches in oncology as there are types of cancer, but the oncologist who treated Roxane taught me two fundamental things. The first, which he learned from another professor: "The cancer cell can do anything to escape the immune system or therapies, and if it doesn't yet know how, it learns very quickly." The second, from himself: "All so-called miraculous remedies are auspicious when used at the right time, with the perspective of changing course if the evolution is not conclusive."

It was a few years after establishing a bridge between traditional Chinese medicine and conventional oncology that I invited this oncologist to give a seminar to my students on addressing the side effects of oncology treatments. I also intervened in the seminar for an afternoon. He appreciated my conclusions, and the seminar was beneficial for everyone. This collaboration, known as "integrative medicine," deepened my humility toward this autoimmune disease. It demands a deeper understanding of its metabolism, stem cells, its interaction with the tissues it exploits, the immune system, and the psyche. Science emphasizes more or less standardized protocols. But from a holistic perspective, each cancer is unique. There is no recipe. The treatment evolves at each stage of the support process.

The final step, when it happens, is healing. However, armed with the experience of the first time, the body is capable of repeating it. Humans fear the day they meet the Grim Reaper, but cancer patients are pursued by it. They must create distance.

Today, Valérie is well; she keeps her distance from cancer. And I'm pleased to see that my need for recognition from my father allowed me to complete this loop of understanding about this disease, that will soon affect, according to World Health Organization (WHO), one out of two people. One loop bumps into another, and so on. The universe of one being is touched by the loop of another, without being able to name what has truly allowed this contact. Carl Jung would tell us that eighty percent of our actions are conditioned by our unconscious mind. In agreement with this concept, my therapeutic direction is to discover with the patient how they will generate their own resolution by illuminating their unique loop. From there, cancer becomes a vessel upon which the patient and their entire therapeutic support progress toward healing.

Throughout life, we all produce numerous cancer cells; some become a part of our biology, while others are relegated to oblivion.

*****

*The force within each of us
is our greatest healer.*
—Hippocrates

My name is Cécile. My mother was diagnosed with Stage 3 ovarian cancer. A wave of panic seized me the morning when I learned that she was receiving gynecological test results. She had been complaining of abdominal pain for several months. The cancer had already spread to the peritoneum. When the diagnosis came, it wasn't the therapist in me who felt it most, but the daughter, with all my helplessness and the range of emotions that accompany a mortal realization. "You can't be the therapist for your own family," they say, just as it's true that a doctor can't be responsible for treating their loved ones. So, I immediately contacted the only holistic therapist experienced with cancer that I knew, Stephen Baudin. Stephen invited me to assist him during his treatments. While sharing some techniques with me, he allowed me to reclaim my role as a caregiver around the massage table that welcomed my mother's body and her suffering. It was a precious gift to be able to rely on another holistic professional like Stephen for her care, while still having an active role in the healing process.

Before my mother was diagnosed, I had spent over fifteen years exploring the world in search of ancestral and traditional natural medicines. I had embarked on this quest for myself to answer existential questions that had been with me since childhood. I lived years learning about healing from shamans, healers, and spiritual leaders. So how could I stand idle? What's the point of all this research if I can't use this knowledge and my practice of energy healing for my own mother? In the role of a daughter, I learned to manage my emotions and to refrain from providing care when my own batteries needed recharging; although, I confess, in some critical moments, I couldn't hold back tears as my eyes gazed upon my mother's emaciated face, her bald head cradled in the dome of my hands. Today, I still provide care for my mother, who has been fighting with unexpected courage for over four years! Meanwhile, she continues to consult Stephen, who has become my husband since then. It was my mother's cancer that brought us together for life!

There are several ways to perceive the body in its energetic dimension: the magnetic grid (energy field or aura) and its various layers, the energy centers (Sanskrit chakras), the channels (Sanskrit nadis), the internal breaths (Sanskrit prana or chi). Each of these serves as gateways that allow me to dive into the unique universe of each patient, to connect with the flow of energy, and to shed light on what requires healing. The energetic dimension serves as an interface between the most subtle realms—spiritual, mental, emotional—and the more physical and chemical realms—organs, tissues, glands, et cetera. Operating from this interface makes contact with all active spheres in the disease.

According to the energetic understanding, the cause of diseases first arises in the subtlest fields and gradually descends to materialize and manifest the illness in the body. It's not uncommon that after radiation or chemotherapy treatments, the patient's energetic grid is damaged, presenting holes or vibrational disturbances in certain areas. While not necessarily painful, this impedes the clear circulation of information and can sabotage the healing process by preventing physical structures from restructuring or regenerating. By restoring harmony in the magnetic grid, the patient's vital energy and self-healing capacities can flow freely and direct themselves according to their own intelligence, exactly where the body needs it in the present moment. By placing hands on specific areas affected by the disease and directing healing energy there, the gentle warmth of touch already provides comfort and encourages the process. What cries out inside the body and mind is like a small child in need of being heard, reassured, and comforted. It's about reclaiming those areas of the body that have been afflicted. Opening the discussion about these questions, how the patient perceives themselves in roles such as mother, lover, or woman, is an integral part of the healing process.

While illness is generally a painful ordeal, it also offers a proposition for intimate and personal evolution. It can reveal itself as an opportunity for self-return. It offers the rare chance to regather, to shine light on all facets of life, and to assess what needs to be abandoned and what needs to be nurtured. It's an inner journey to mobilize, to dare to confront, and to trust one's own destiny in conditions that invite both death and life. Thanks to this return to oneself, the patient accesses spaces within that they may never have inhabited or that seem deserted by benevolence and love. In this sense, energy healing facilitates sudden realizations that encourage achievable and beneficial changes in the patient's life, thereby supporting their healing.

Tammy Rader
Embracing the journey

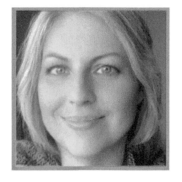

Tammy Rader is a contributor to and two-time International Best-Selling author of *The Cinderella Monologues* and *Live Life in W.O.W! Nuggets of Wonder, Openness & Wisdom*, and is an emerging speaker.

She is a cancer survivor and mentor, focused on guiding those with cancer through and beyond their journey to triumph.

Having been diagnosed just 39 days apart with both breast and rectal cancer, Tammy is now a "Thriver", who finds resilience with the help of humor, a practicing mindset, and having gratitude.

Tammy currently lives in Edmonton, Alberta, Canada. She is the Founder of *BeYOUtiful Beyond Your Diagnosis (by Tam)* and offers Nurture Mail (cards), journals, programs, group coaching, and 1:1 talks.

She loves the simple little things in life, like going for walks, the sound of laughter, ladybugs, unicorns, and flip flops.

Website: www.beyoutiful.health

Email: Tammy@beyoutiful.health

LinkedIn: linkedin.com/in/tammyrader

Facebook: facebook.com/tammy.rader.35

Instagram: instagram.com/tammy.rader73

Tammy Rader
Embracing the journey

In the middle of difficulty, lies opportunity.
—Albert Einstein

"I love you" are three little words everyone wants to hear. Three devastating words no one wants to hear are "You have cancer." Unfortunately, I heard those words twice—just thirty-nine days apart!

After hearing those words, I am grateful to be "here" and to share my story! I'm not sure that I would be, though, without the help of a strong mindset, gratitude (stubbornness), and the ability to find humor in it all. Yes, humor in having cancer.

I grew up in a very small town, Dashwood, Ontario, Canada. I had the most extraordinary, loving, kind parents. They celebrated their fiftieth wedding anniversary in 2020! Sadly, just fourteen days shy of their fifty-second anniversary, my dad passed away. My parents had two children: me (the best one first), then my brother three years later.

I have one son, Steven, whom I call my "little man." Steven is a miracle because, at age sixteen, I was diagnosed with endometriosis and irritable bowel syndrome (IBS). I was told I would never have children. But several years and laseroscopies later (surgeries to clean out the endometriosis), I found out I was pregnant! Steven has grown into a fine young man whom I am very proud of! He works hard at his full-time job and creates custom woodworking. He's made some beautiful pieces, but the most precious piece he's made in my eyes is the one-of-a-kind piece he made for me.

Steven's dad and I ended up in a nasty divorce when Steven was eight years old. It caused a great deal of stress for all of us. (Today we are friends). After the divorce, I took on more jobs and worked hard. I took the necessary steps to demonstrate and teach my son that no matter what life deals you, you must show up and never give up!

On a Monday morning in January 2021, I had just gotten out of the shower. I grazed my chest as I was combing my long dark hair. That felt weird. I looked at myself in the mirror, did a quick self-exam, and I found a rather large lump in my right breast. My heart skipped a beat and I thought, I'm working too hard. I've carried boxes that were too heavy. I've been stressed. Yes, that's it! It's cancer! NO, that's NOT it! Wait!! No one in my family has had breast cancer! I dismissed the thought and carried on.

I let things go for a week and checked again. The lump was still there. I called my doctor, who ordered a mammogram and ultrasound, which led to biopsies. I told myself it was nothing...but deep down I knew.

In the middle of a February afternoon, while I was at work, I received a phone call. I saw the doctor's number—I didn't have an appointment. Chills went through me before I answered. My doctor confirmed my worst thoughts. "You have cancer."

She said so much more to me, but when I heard "those" words, none of her other words made sense.

Next, the surgeon called, and he explained I had an aggressive form of breast cancer as it had already spread to my lymph nodes under my arm. I had to have a single mastectomy.

What the hell was happening? I felt a huge blow to my gut! The tears came immediately! What am I going to look like? What will others say or think? How is this going to affect my relationship with my partner, David? Will he still love me? So many things!!

I had to call my family, who live 3,000 miles away. Those were the worst phone calls I've ever had to make! So many tears, so many questions, with no answers.

When I woke from my mastectomy, I had a blue binding on and two tubes protruding from my right side. Surgeons had taken my right breast and seventeen lymph nodes from my armpit. If that weren't bad enough... two weeks after the mastectomy, before staples were removed, I heard those devastating words again! "You have cancer." This time it came from a gastroenterologist.

Earlier, I mentioned that most of my life I've had IBS and endometriosis. I've also had multiple surgeries to my gut, including a hysterectomy and an appendectomy. In 2017, I was in a car accident and another in 2018—neither accident my fault, just to clarify. In 2019, I sensed "things" weren't right. I was in a lot of pain. I had been constipated my whole life but it was going to new "levels." Back to the doctor. A colonoscopy was booked for April of 2020—and we all know what happened in 2020—a pandemic. And surprise! My appointment was canceled, twice, ultimately pushing the colonoscopy back to thirty-nine days after my breast cancer diagnosis and fourteen days after my mastectomy.

Sitting in the GI specialist's office with David, waiting for the results, my stomach was in a knot. You know that feeling in the pit of your gut when something isn't right? That's what I felt. The doctor came in and looked at me. I could see it in his eyes. I asked him—begged him not to say the words. But he did. "I'm sorry. I don't have good news."

I said, "NO, please!"

He said, "I'm sorry, you have rectal cancer."

I lost it! Another blow to the gut! I started crying, sobbing. Through my tears, I asked, "How could this be happening again?"

David came over and held me. He had tears in his eyes too. I thought, What the hell am I going to do now? Most people hear those words once in a lifetime and some hear those words for a second or third time, if the cancer comes back, but geez, to hear those same words SO close together was an absolute nightmare!!

When you are faced with those words, so many thoughts cross your mind—death being one—and questions. How much time do I have? Am I going to die? How the hell am I going to tell my family? And I thought the first call I made to them about the breast cancer was the worst call. Guess again. This one was worse!!

As I was having my staples removed from my first surgery, the mastectomy, a few days later, I realized I **can** do hard things! Did I want to do hard things? No. Who does? But I wasn't going down without a fight! Death was not an option because my "want" to live was so great! My mom has always said, "They broke the mold when they made you." She'd agree, I am stubborn and a fighter! My attitude, perseverance, and resilience will get me through this!

Breast treatments had to be put on hold, and we started treatments for the rectal cancer first. Welcome, thirty-six radiation treatments and three rounds of chemo. I had thought radiation was a "bad sunburn." It's not! It is the worst sunburn you can get, and you burn from the inside out. I lost four layers of skin from my pubic bone to my tailbone and inside my thighs. I couldn't walk right for almost six weeks and the pain! UUGGHH! I was so awesome at handling these treatments that my reward was a prolapsed bladder (eyeroll).

Due to the pandemic and restrictions on travel, it had been over two years since I had seen my family. Between my treatments, I was granted permission to fly from my home in Alberta to Ontario. By this time, I was losing my hair. Thanks, chemo! You know, it's funny. I was more scared of losing my hair than I was of having the chemo! People will say, "It's just hair. It'll grow back." No!! It's not just hair! Please do not say this to someone who is going through chemo or to someone who is losing their hair for any other reason! (Some people lose their hair to cancer and it doesn't grow back!! Don't even get me started on "Now you can get a free boob job!" Just don't say it!)

Cancer takes so damn much from you. I wanted to take control! I needed to! Cancer had to know—I am the boss of me! I wanted to feel empowered!

I asked my son, "Will you help me shave my head?" He looked at me and without hesitation, he said, "Yeah, I'll even shave mine!" I felt so much love at that moment! I put the hair I had left into a ponytail and he cut it off. After that, six of us took turns shaving my head. It was an incredible, empowering, beautiful moment. I still get choked up when I think about it—I took control! I didn't let cancer take that from me. And it turns out, I *looked pretty good bald!*

Back in Alberta, I started treatments for my breast cancer. Welcome six rounds of chemo and twenty radiation treatments. Chemo challenged my body. Each time, I ended up in the hospital. One time, it was for five days! I had zero immune system! That was the scariest time of this journey. I didn't know if I would be coming home!

Funny story (not really), one time I was administered too much chemo. Chemo is mixed specifically for the patient, considering age, height, weight, and type of cancer. The stage and grade all matter and go into the concoction. They got it right for the next dose!

I finished my last chemo treatment in November 2021 and **all** my treatments by February 2022! I rang my third and final bell (most people only ring one bell), signaling this part of the journey was over. Then it was on to healing, recouping, and learning to live my best life for the rest of my life!

At least that's what I thought.

When life is supposed to "go back to normal," you're left with a slew of side effects, trying to process a bunch of emotions, all while attempting to pick up the pieces of your life and "move on" without really knowing how to integrate this into your life. It sucks! Believe me. The system isn't set up for you after treatments! The medical system is amazing for treating cancer—and I'm very grateful for the care I received—but it's not designed to support your longevity, mental or emotional health, and it falls short in terms of post-treatment preventative care.

Fast forward one year (plus) post treatments. I had a major roller-coaster ride of health issues. From neuropathy in my fingers and toes to chemo brain—it's friggin' real!! As a result of a prolapsed bladder and radiation, I had major kidney infections, way too many hospital "visits," severe fatigue, nausea—and the list goes on! As I'm sure you can guess by now, I'm not one that "sugar coats" things. I tell it like it is. And it's not all sunshine, rainbows, and unicorns after treatment is over!

Complaining doesn't solve problems—gratitude, on the other hand, can help. Gratitude creates the mindset you need to find opportunity everywhere, despite negative, challenging, and overwhelming circumstances. Did you know, grateful people are attractive, fascinating, and magnetic? Well, now you do! Have a look around and see what you can consciously be grateful for!

I don't normally talk about private things (who am I kidding), but the very first time I showered after my first surgery—"first" because twenty-two months after my first mastectomy, I had my second mastectomy (And last! What more can they take?)—the shower was hard! I still had staples in and a thin bandage over them, but medical staff allowed me to shower because the nurse was coming to change bandages. I stood under the warm running water and for a second, it felt good, "normal." Then I realized—I could feel the warm water on my collar bone and on my stomach. But I could not feel the water, not just where the ten-and-a-half inch (yes, I measured it) scar was across my chest, but all around it and part of my underarm. What the heck was going on? I was numb! I started to cry. I stood there, in the shower, and sobbed. Why was I not told this was a feeling (or lack thereof) I would experience? Why was I not told this was going to be a moment of "pain," grief, and sadness for the loss of my breast? Then I felt anger. Why me? Why did this happen to me? So many thoughts go through your mind! Standing there with the water running, it hit me. Not everyone in this world gets to have clean, warm running water. Not everyone gets the medical attention I was given.

Then gratitude started and I thought ... Why NOT me?

One of the hardest things you will ever face is finding self-love/acceptance for your body after a lumpectomy, mastectomy (or two), or whatever surgery you've had. The changes to your body are *not just physical* but emotional as well. I am still working on acceptance and finding self-love for my new body. At first, it was hard to look in the mirror and see that person standing in front of me! It took some work (journalling, counselling, mantras, affirmations), and I was able to reflect on, and feel gratitude for, the strength of my body. I took baby steps forward and started to embrace this new person in the mirror. As time went on, seeing beyond the physical, making small mental shifts, I started nurturing my body from within. The biggest realization for me was that it's okay to look different! Whatever "different" looks like for you.

Gratitude and humor played a huge part here! Yes, I said humor. If you've read to here, I'm sure you've caught some of my sarcastic remarks/thoughts about this journey so far. Laughter is a medicine and it costs nothing! Watching funny animal videos, people-falling videos, listening to your favorite comedian, or having simple conversations with your friends/family and laughing together—that's the best medicine of all! Going through a diagnosis (or something difficult) and learning to laugh at yourself is the best gift!

There are so many more things I could talk about, like some of the "dark moments." The nights I stayed up as long as I could because I was so scared, if I fell asleep, I wouldn't wake up. Or the days I would cry from the pain, nausea, or the dreaded thoughts of what's coming next. I tried to not stay in those "dark moments" for long, and eventually I found some "tools" to help me cope, like, it's okay to grieve what you've lost! The loss of a body part, whether you have reconstruction or choose to stay flat like I did, doesn't matter—it's a grieving process!

Here are a few things that helped me:

- Remember, the only healthy and worthwhile comparison is the person you were yesterday versus the person you are today. Focus on that!

- Ask yourself, what can I find to be grateful for today? Even if it's just the fact that you woke up!

- "Pivot don't panic." If you want to sit in a chair and stare at a wall, do it, but set a timer for fifteen minutes and then get up, go for a walk, take a nap or a bubble bath, read a book, or call a friend. Cut out the crap that's too much for you, but also move forward, even if it's baby steps!

Going back to the thought, "Why NOT me?" Why not embrace the journey and find all the **opportunities** that you can! I have met extraordinary people through my journey and done extraordinary things. I am working on my own book and had the privilege to be a contributing author in two anthologies, making me a two-time, international bestselling author. I won a trip to California with a friend who also had cancer. I am now an *After Breast Cancer Ambassador* and I get to have a photoshoot and be in a calendar. My point is, ask yourself, What am I learning about myself? and tell yourself, Never let a good disaster go to waste! It may not seem like it in certain moments, but always remember: Life is f*cking good!

You don't have to have cancer to feel like crap. You don't always feel like crap when you have cancer. You **do** have to have tools and clarity to move yourself forward and that's where "BeYOUtiful Beyond Your Diagnosis" comes in.

BeYOUtiful is a safe, comfortable, and interactive online support community for any point during your cancer journey. You are BeYOUtiful in every moment throughout the highs, lows, and everything in between. There is still a bright future ahead of your diagnosis, and I'm here to help you find it! Reach out if you need help or just want to talk.

Oh, wait! I want to tell you about that custom, one-of-a-kind piece my son, Steven, made for me. It's a large, thick chunk of live edge wood (the bark is still on it). He planed it down to super smooth and carved a cancer ribbon in the middle of it. He filled the ribbon with two colors of epoxy (blue and pink for rectal and breast cancer). In the very middle at the top of the ribbon, he inserted half of my staples from my mastectomy (my idea—a total of thirty staples). He placed them in the shape of a heart. He also incorporated lights in it. It's the most beautiful gift I have ever received! Steven is my whole world and one of the many reasons I fought (and still fight) for my life!

Cancer may have started this fight, but I'm going to finish it!

Tracey Downing
Little did I know

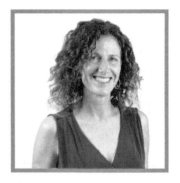

Tracey Downing has dedicated her life's journey to empowering individuals to discover newfound confidence in their physical abilities and take command of their long-term well-being. Together with her husband, she established a health promotion company in 2000, impacting numerous lives by guiding them towards positive lifestyle shifts and instilling the importance of prioritizing their health.

Her academic journey at the University of Michigan, where she graduated with a degree in Kinesiology, was complemented by a vibrant period of exploration. Tracey's adventures took her across the globe to places like New Zealand, Ireland, and Scotland. These enriching experiences allowed her to indulge her passion for travel while simultaneously nurturing her professional growth, with roles in clinical and professional sports settings.

Beyond her entrepreneurial pursuits, Tracey treasures her role as a mother to two wonderful children. Outside of her business endeavors, she has completed an Ironman Triathlon, a testament to her unwavering determination, and she had the incredible honor of being an Olympic Torch Bearer for the Salt Lake City Olympics.

In Tracey's world, fostering physical wellness is not just a profession, it's a lifelong vocation driven by a genuine desire to inspire and uplift others on their unique journeys toward lasting health and vitality.

Instagram: Tracey-Downing

FaceBook: traceydowning

Tracey Downing
Little did I know

I believe the circles of women around
us weave invisible nets of love that
carry us when we are weak and sing
with us when we are strong.
—Sark

I miss hugging—the feeling of sinking into someone and feeling them sink into me. See, I had a double mastectomy thirteen years ago and of all the losses I prepared myself for, this was not among them. I was twenty-nine when I was diagnosed with a highly aggressive form of breast cancer. I had just completed my first Ironman triathlon, was about to close on our first house, and was planning for my wedding, a few months away at the time. I was riding the high of accomplishment, proud of myself, impressed by the ability of my mind and body to endure, excited about all that was to come. My diagnosis put an end to that pretty darn quick. My body had betrayed me. I went from a celebratory state to one of survival.

While shocking, this, unfortunately, was not the start of what's become my lifelong entanglements with breast cancer. My mother was diagnosed when I was nine years old, then again when I was eleven. This was in the early 1980s before breast cancer awareness was even a thing. Back then, cancer was spoken about in whispers. For me, at nine years old, it was downright terrifying. My mom had a single mastectomy at the time. She was thirty-six. The recurrence happened as she was going through the breast expansion process and the radiation therapy that ensued led to a contracture. Young and beautiful, at age thirty-eight, for all intent and purpose, my mom's reconstruction failed and her experience of hugs, perhaps like mine, was forever altered.

Myriad genetics found and patented the BRCA1 gene (a/k/a the breast cancer gene) in 1994. I was twenty-one years old, a sophomore in college and my older sister was preparing to apply to business school. My mother's doctor did not feel there was a need for my mother, nor my sister and I to be tested. As my mother was the first case of breast cancer in our family tree, he was not concerned. We all breathed a sigh of relief.

I knew I was supposed to do self-exams but, if I'm being honest, I was not particularly vigilant about them. Somewhere in the recesses of my mind lingered a belief that I would someday be diagnosed, but "someday" felt very far away at twenty-one years of age.

That is until a typical afternoon a few weeks after Ironman when I was changing clothes after a workout. As I performed the contortions required to get out of my sports bra, my fingers grazed a lump that I hadn't noticed before. I consulted doctors about it, but they clearly didn't expect a healthy twenty-nine-year-old in great shape to present with breast cancer. No mammogram was ordered, no ultrasound, no MRI. I was sent home with a recommendation to use hot compresses and triple antibiotic ointment.

With the lump still there after following the doctor's recommendation for a few weeks, I returned and asked if it could be removed. While this request likely saved my life, I felt like a hypochondriac. My doctor couldn't have been less alarmed even though I told her about my family history. The surgeon she referred me to explained that it wasn't cancer, but if I was worried about it, he would remove it. Even my mother, after hearing how laissez-faire both doctors were, explained that just because she had had cancer, didn't mean I had to have every lump and bump removed. I didn't even bother to mention it to my father, nor to my sister.

A week or so later, I drove myself to outpatient surgery for a procedure that would be performed under local anesthesia. So convinced was my surgeon that this was nothing, the surgical consent form read "removal of a nodule, right axilla." The word "biopsy" was nowhere to be seen. When I asked if it would be sent for pathology, the surgeon explained that he had to send it out; otherwise, my insurance would consider the procedure cosmetic.

It's been twenty years and I have yet to understand the arrogance of these two doctors.

In the days and weeks that followed, my fiancé and I set about learning as much as we could and putting together our dream team in terms of care providers. Thankfully, we live in Silicon Valley with easy access to world-class medical institutions. I was quickly referred to genetic oncology and Stanford's Tumor Board. On my fiancé's thirty-seventh birthday, my sister came with me to Tumor Board where they confirmed what we suspected ... that I carried the BRCA1 genetic mutation. Not only did this have lifelong implications for me, but it also put what we thought was my mother's minimal cancer risk in question, as well as my sister's.

What it meant for me was that, out of the gates, all specialties represented at Tumor Board agreed that the best course of action was prophylactic bilateral mastectomies, followed by chemo and possibly radiation. We knew this was likely should the genetic result come back as it did, but that didn't make it any less of a bomb being dropped on my life. The doctors were kind and patient, but none acknowledged that the surgery would likely leave me without feeling in my breasts, that it was obviously not going to be possible for me to breastfeed future children, as I had imagined up until a few weeks earlier, and that, if I followed the recommended course, a hug would never feel the same. In the doctors' minds, this was life-saving surgery. In mine, this was an irreversible, life-altering surgery. I'd gone from planning for my future, starting with my wedding, to worrying if I would have one. I first opted for a lumpectomy, as that was a decision I could, and eventually did, reverse; but at that moment in time, cancer had taken so much, I wasn't willing to give it any more than was absolutely necessary.

Roughly two months following that meeting with Tumor Board, having had the lumpectomy, eggs harvested, embryos frozen, and four rounds of dose-dense chemo completed, me and my bald head walked down the aisle. While I did not have the typical pre-wedding checklist, I didn't have time to mourn that; I was too busy taking every step I could to ensure my future. Our "wigs optional" wedding was quite a celebration. Returning home to chemo rather than boarding a plane to our Fijian honeymoon not so much! However, little more than a year after my Tumor Board meeting, six months after completing treatment, we learned we were pregnant.

If my diagnosis was a betrayal, my pregnancy was redemption. Having been through all that it had, my body had made a miraculous recovery even though my spirit seemed to be lagging behind. My life appeared back on track with cancer having been a temporary detour. Except that's not really how it works, is it?

I recall looking in the mirror and feeling like I was looking at a stranger. Having had curly hair my whole life, I was more than familiar with the painstaking process of growing out my curly locks. That didn't make it any more pleasant. I didn't look like myself and I definitely didn't feel like myself. Add pregnancy changes and hormones to the mix and it's probably not a stretch to imagine that I was a bit of a wreck. I was relieved and genuinely grateful to have become pregnant, but happiness was an emotion that I couldn't quite put my hands on.

We moved into our new home while I was going through treatment, having closed on the purchase within days of my diagnosis. We weren't far from friends, but they weren't right around the corner either. I remember my husband, worried about my emotional state, suggesting I join a mom's group and begin building a community. The thought of meeting new people, the energy from which I typically thrive, was daunting. I believed, given my emotional state, I would not attract the type of people I wanted and needed in my life and felt powerless to change it. Similar to looking in the mirror, this trepidation around meeting and getting to know people was just as foreign. I could put on some makeup and pretend to be lighthearted, fun, and interesting. I was thirty years old, had started my own business four years prior, was an Ironman Triathlete, an Olympic torchbearer, a world traveler ... yet my experience with cancer seemed, unavoidably, to find its way into conversation very quickly in the "get to know you" process. Buzz kill!

It is said that time heals all wounds. Or maybe you just distract yourself with more pressing matters. In my case, our son and our business provided plenty of distraction.

Finding a lump in my breast when I was eight months pregnant with our daughter and four years post-treatment threw me right back into the fray. None of our doctors were overly concerned, but given the process of my initial diagnosis, we weren't eager to take their word for it. Although it turned out to be nothing, my husband and I agreed that, once I was done breastfeeding (yes, I was able to nurse both our children from the non-irradiated side), we would return to doctors, re-hear, and re-evaluate the information on which we based our initial treatment decisions and perhaps reconsider them.

Ultimately, the only new information we received was enough for us to decide to proceed with the prophylactic bilateral mastectomies. We were told that I had already received nearly my lifetime limit of Adriamycin, which at the time was the best drug available to treat my particular cancer. So back we went into the medical establishment to figure out the hows and whens of mastectomy surgery and implant reconstruction. I wrestled with making peace with the decision to proceed. Speaking to our surgeon about the impact to intimacy, he looked straight at my husband and said something to the effect of "That's for you to figure out." Sharing my concerns with my BFF the day before surgery about disfigurement and, perhaps, craziness at having such a massive surgery when I didn't even have cancer, she responded, "Reframe it. Tomorrow, you GET to have lifesaving surgery!" No matter the spin, I was thirty-four years old and my body, as I knew it, would never be the same. And a hug would never feel the same.

A few years later, I was told it was time to think about having my ovaries removed as I was nearing forty. This plan had been explained to me back when I received my genetic results; however, little information was offered as to the question of "then what?" I hadn't had a trace of cancer for nearly ten years, yet somehow it continued to be an unwelcome disruption to my present and my future. This is not to say I hadn't gotten on with my life—my hair had grown back; I was fully engaged in both my personal and professional lives; my marriage and my children were sources of pride and joy. I wouldn't say I worried about the cancer returning, but I never felt like it completely went away either.

Back when my personal journey with cancer began, a friend likened the experience to aging prematurely. Same-aged friends were doing what normal thirty-somethings should be doing, worrying about what normal thirty-some-things should be worried about. I was doing and worrying about many of the same things, just with an added sprinkle of losing my breasts and going through menopause.

As to the question of "then what?" regarding the removal of my ovaries, the cancer world had little to offer. On the wom-en's health side, I got a definitive "not-touching-that-with-a-ten-foot-pole" vibe. Everyone agreed removing my ovaries at thirty-eight was the right thing to do, but no one had answers to questions about my sex life, my bone health, or my quality of life. A compromise was eventually struck: If I had a complete hysterectomy, I could go on complete hormone replacement therapy (HRT), at least until the time I would have naturally gone through menopause. The next hurdle was which hor-mones and at what dose. My oncologist said, "I don't know, I don't prescribe hormones," while my obstetrician—still keep-ing my "situation" at a distance—asked for more specific guid-ance. I am happy to report, we eventually got things figured out and I have been safely under the care of a practitioner who specializes in HRT for many years now.

The best thing about the hysterectomy was that once it was done, nine years after diagnosis, I had finally completed my prevent-cancer checklist. Not exactly a celebratory moment, but at least there was nothing looming in the future. Unfortunately, though, breast cancer wasn't quite as ready to move on from my world as I was for it to do so. Earlier this year, my sister was diagnosed—nineteen years after I was diagnosed, which was twenty years after my mother was diagnosed. As I listened to the information and recommendations my sister was receiving, it was as if no time had passed. It was all too familiar.

I am grateful for the strength and resilience of not only my body but also that of my mother's and sister's. In all of this, the thing that frustrates me most is how quickly the recommendations come to cut out parts of a woman's body without much recognition of or attention to what will be lost. The treatments and recommendations I received were intended for older women—it wasn't my doctors' fault that I happened to be twenty-nine years old at diagnosis. I don't regret any of the decisions we made. I think the world of our care providers. I genuinely believe everything I went through, while maybe not lifesaving, was definitely life-extending. If there is anything I would change, it would be to have grieved the parts of me that I would and did lose rather than trying to tie up the whole experience in a pretty pink ribbon. There are many things that I miss, that were taken by cancer and won't be returned, but a big, smooshy, enveloping, heart-to-heart hug, without the barrier of implants, is at the top of the list.

Sophie Rouméas
About the anthologist

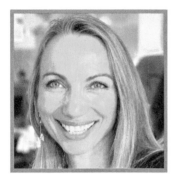

Enthusiastic about the profound impact of words in evoking emotions, memories, and reflection, Sophie Rouméas channels this passion into her therapeutic practice, guiding meditation, hypnosis sessions, and family constellations.

To serve both current and future generations while honoring our ancestors, she launched a three-day online conference featuring international speakers. The conference was dedicated to sharing techniques and methods for healing the family tree.

Sophie compiled and published a first anthology, J'ai vécu la même chose que toi, written with twelve co-authors and available in French. The best-seller testifies to the resilience displayed by these young women who recovered from breast cancer as a message of hope and encouragement for the families affected by this ordeal. Creating *Angel Lab Editions* and publishing collective books on sensitive topics like breast cancer with committed and concerned co-authors, aligns with one of Sophie's strong values, out of solidarity.

Born in the French Alps, nature has consistently fueled Sophie's creativity, inspiring intuition, attentiveness, and self-expression in others. Her guiding motto in her work is: *Let's voice your soul!*

Mother of Maxime and Donovan, Sophie lovingly bridges her family and community in both France and California, where her partner Sam resides with his family.

sophie.roumeas@gmail.com

Individual sessions: www.sophieroumeas.com

Family Tree: www.healingthefamilytree.com

www.facebook.com/sophie.roumeas1/

Books:

J'ai vécu la même chose que toi

Souls in Love

GRATITUDE

Dear readers,

This anthology began with the intention of uniting voices to enhance our understanding of the challenges presented by breast cancer. We extend our profound gratitude to our authors for their authenticity and invaluable testimonials. Each and every one of them has allowed the magic of solidarity, both individually and collectively, to be interwoven for those for whom this book is dedicated.

We warmly thank our loved ones, families, friends, communities, and cherished allies in life who guide us toward connecting with our hearts, fostering comprehension and compassion, and embodying healing, care, sharing, receiving, and giving back. Ultimately, these experiences lead us towards a state of positive and proactive unity.

For the narratives:

The 14 authors

For the editing/proofreading of chapters and bios:

Kay Clark-Uhle

For the interior layout and design, the launch preparation and support, and her powerful smile:

Rebecca Hall Gruyter and her team with RHG Medias Productions

For the book cover design:

Darko Dojchinovski

For the head shot of Crystal Weber:

Photo credit © Jérôme Gorin

We will gratefully welcome your comments, reviews, or simply hearing from you at hello@pinkandunited.org

Yours sincerely,

Sophie Rouméas

on behalf of the Angel Lab Editions team

Made in the USA
Las Vegas, NV
22 November 2023

81359132R00095